LEAN AND GREEN COOKBOOK

1000-Day Easy and Yummy Recipes to Eat
Well Everyday and Lose Weight Fast without
Feeling on a Diet | Discover the Secrets
of the "Fuelings Hacks Meal"!

by

Lara Ward

Click here to get 10 EXTRA Lean and Green Recipes for FREE! :

https://bit.ly/3tSipRd

Table of Contents

INTRODUCTION

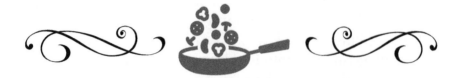

THE BASICS OF LEAN AND GREEN DIET

A lean and green meal consists of 5 to 7 ounces of cooked magic protein plus three portions of non-starchy and two portions of healthy fats, depending on your choice of lean proteins. You can enjoy your Lean & Green meals for any of your six meals all day long or whatever works best on your food schedule.

Lean and green food offers essential calories, healthy fats, protein, fiber and other nutrients that differ from our foodstuffs' nutritional composition. Take the healthy fat component of the green and lean food, for instance. Add a daily dose of healthy fat to your meal plan is important because it helps your body absorb vitamins such as A, D, E, and K and help your gallbladder work properly.

The lean and green meal also provides the right calorie, carbohydrate and protein balance to fuel your body while promoting a mild but efficient fat burning condition. The meal also offers volume to keep you comfortable and satisfied.

A lean and green meal is an opportunity to learn how to make healthy, nutritious meals for you and your family.

Weight loss benefits, how does it work?

A slimmer body is the most visible sign of weight loss. However, there are many important changes, including the following ones that you cannot see.

1. **Heartburn reduced**: - Extra pounds put pressure on your belly, which can cause acid to flow into your esophagus and cause a heartburn's fiery discomfort. The opposite is true: weight loss reduces pressure and burns down.

2. **Reduced pain in the knee**: - we all know it is the leg that lifts or carries the body's weight. You put about 4 pounds of stress on the knee joints per additional pound. For a person with a weight of 150 pounds (10 pounds and a weight of 140 pounds), the extra 10 pounds add 40 more pounds of pressure each step. But he would relieve 30 pounds of pressure with a total weight loss of 5% to reduce the weight he places on his knees and feet.

3. **Blood pressure decreased**. For adults with excess weight, the risk of high blood pressure triples. But each pound of weight loss can lead to a one-point decrease in both your blood pressure measurement numbers, upper (systolic) and lower (diastolic). This would be a drop in blood pressure of almost eight points for a 150 pound person with a 5% loss of body weight.

4. **Reduced risk of diabetes**: -Weight gain is a strong risk factor for diabetes development.

*Fat is not only a passive calorie storage site. Adipokines, known as adipogenic chemicals which are secreted by fatty cells, can cause inflammation, and interfere with insulin's action; more fat, more adipokines; But weight loss reduces adipokines, reduces blood sugar levels by insulin and reduces the risk of diabetes; "**Says Dr. David M. Nathan, director of the Harvard Massachusetts***

General Hospital Diabetes Center and Clinical Research Centre.

1. **Improved sexual function**: -Overweight and obesity can decrease sexual function and improve recovery of healthy weight. The reason is that a healthy weight lowers blood pressure and stops diabetes, and sex can interfere with both high blood pressure and diabetes.

2. **Sleep improved**: -People with excess weight may have obstructive sleep apnea, a poor sleep condition characterized by many nighttime breathing pauses. *"The loss of weight often reduces sleep apnea and restores sleep," Dr. Stanford says.*

3. **Extra power and body Energy:** -The more weight you gain, the more difficult it is for your body to work. This requires more adenosine triphosphate (ATP)— the molecule that supplies cells with energy. If you lose weight, you use less ATP so that you have more energy.

4. **Increased self-appreciation**:- "Weight is linked to self-esteem for some people. They feel better, interact more with others and feel good about life when they lose weight, "Medical Doctors.

5. How Does Weight Loss works:-

• Eat right: -"Eat lean proteins, whole grains, fruit, vegetables, nuts and seeds. Concentrate on a healthy diet rather than just the amount of calories you consume.

• Exercise: -Target for moderate intensity activity for at least 150 minutes per week. That might mean walking for many older adults, if you can't go out, or it may mean marching, walking side by side, or dancing, and using music to speed up or slow down your pace. It makes weight loss patients feel helpful and healthy.

- Get enough sleep. "Weight-regulating brain pathways interact with pathways which regulate sleep," Try to get regular and consistent sleep, it helps keep your weight loss healthy.

What you should eat and what to avoid.

Heavily processed foods can make it difficult to maintain a steady loss of weight, but some of the best foods for weight loss are those high in fiber. Fibrous foods are often lower in calories, help you stay satiated following a meal, and regulate your blood sugar levels. Research suggests that the more dietary fiber you integrate into your daily life, the more you can fight "abdominal fat deposits."

You can lose weight and naturally reduce body fat by taking a healthy diet along with moderate exercise. It's important to eliminate processed foods high in sodium and other succulents because they stay routinely hydrated to support digestion, and to keep track of your overall effort to lose weight.

Healthy eating and weight loss can be connected to the consumption of the following kind of foods:-

1. Tuna
2. Chickpeas
3. Salmon
4. Pumpkin
5. Potatoes
6. Walnut
7. Almond
8. Peanut Butter
9. Asparagus
10. Cruciferous Vegetables
11. Lean beef and chicken breast

Fruits that help in weight loss can include:-

1. Avocado
2. Grapefruit
3. Rhubarb
4. Apple

5. Kiwi Fruit
6. Banana
7. Berries
8. Orange
9. Stone Fruit
10. Melons
11. Passion Fruit

Foods you should avoid when losing weight:-

1. Sugary Drinks
2. Pastries, cookies and cakes
3. French Fries and Chips
4. Alcohol (Especially Beer)
5. High calories drinks
6. Food high in sugar content
7. Candy Bars
8. Fruit Juices
9. Baked foods
10. Pasta and Bread

Common mistakes and difficulties you will encounter while trying to lose weight:-

1. Choosing products for 'diet.'

Storing your dietary food is one of the surest ways to fail in your mission of weight loss. Make dietary products your priority and instead fill your diet with whole-food, vegetable-based foods.

2. Stop starving your belly

While a dramatic reduction of calories and a quick fix for weight loss may seem like a skipped meal, under-eating can actually sabotage your effort to shed these extra pounds.

While it is an efficient way to lose weight to consume fewer calories than you consume, a sharp and dramatic reduction in calories can cause your body to hunger. If this happens, your metabolism slows into a crawling, slow-burning calorie to conserve its energy store. That is why people who too often cut out too many reach a point where you stop losing weight.

Lose of weight seldom happens quickly nor is it easy to achieve sustainable results. Rather than wanting a quick solution, adopt the motto 'race wins slow and steady.' This means that calories are reduced to a sensitive level and a weight-loss objective of 1-2 pounds per week is set.

3. Cutting out whole food groups

Many popular fad diets teach people to cut off whole food groups, such as fats and carbs.

Carbohydrates were crucified as a key cause for weight gain and no-carb diets became all too common. Although refined carbohydrates such as sugar and white bread may spike blood glucose and cause weight gain, complex carbohydrates such as a grain of rice can contribute to weight loss.

The risks of developing nutrient deficiencies, such as fiber or protein, are also a major concern to eliminate whole food groups. If you have no real food allergy, be careful to embark on a weight loss scheme that requires you to say important healthy staples.

So, Instead of removing entire food groups, try to swap certain unhealthy elements for healthier alternatives. Top Tip: Replace white bread, pasta and rice with wholegrain counterparts, for example, and swap unhealthy fats with avocados and nuts in processed foods.

The Mistake of too many or too few calories consumption

For weight loss, a calorie deficit is required. This means that you have more calories to burn than you consume.You may feel like you don't eat a lot of calories. However, most of us tend to underestimate and underestimate what we eat.

You may eat too many healthy and highly calorific foods like noodles and cheese, but it is important to watch your portion sizes.On the other hand, too much decreasing your calorie consumption can be counterproductive.

1. Excessive Exercising

If you don't do anything while calories are being limited, you will probably lose more muscle weight and decrease metabolic rates.

In contrast, exercise minimizes the slender mass you lose, increases your fat loss and prevents slowing down your metabolism. The slighter you have, the easier it is to lose weight and keep weight.

Over-exercise, however, also leads to a problem of stress. It is likened that you are trying to force your body to use too many calories that are neither effective nor healthy. It may also affect the production of adrenal hormones that regulate stress response.

2. Avoiding the consumption of Protein

It is very important to get enough protein if you try to lose weight. Protein has been shown to help in a number of ways with weight loss. It can reduce appetite, increase fullness, reduce calorie intake, improve metabolism, and protect muscle mass during the loss of weight. So, avoiding protein that it might add to your weight is not advisable, it is even very important.

Higher protein diets can benefit the control of appetite and body composition. Make sure that every meal contains a high protein food to optimize weight loss. High protein intake helps reduce appetite, increases sensations of fullness and increases the rate of metabolism.

3. Restraining yourself from Sleep

Sleep deprivation causes changes in our appetite and hunger hormones. The hormone is produced less due to bad sleep and it reduces your food appetite and promotes energy in the body.It affects the food you want and can stimulate intense cravings for foods rich in fat and sugar.

Your brain struggles after poor sleep to make the best judgment about food, so you are more likely to be impulsive and give up to unhealthy food hunger.Make sure you sleep in total darkness to improve your sleep quanta and quality while avoiding a few hours of blue light from mobile phones and devices.

Now, that we have exposed you to the different sections of weight loss practices, it's expedient for us to give you the limitless list of vegan recipes (or lean and green meals) that you must embrace to help your healthy weight loss journey.

Sit back and enjoy!

BREAKFAST RECIPES

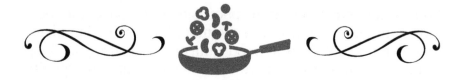

SKINNY GREEN CHILE CHICKEN ENCHILADA DIP

YIELD: 4 Servings

PER SERVING: 1 Lean, ½ Green, 1 Healthy Fat, 3 Condiment

INGREDIENTS:

- 4 ounces low-fat cream cheese, room temperature
- 1 cup plain low-fat Greek yogurt
- ¼ cup green enchilada sauce
- 7-ounce dice green chillies
- ½ tsp cumin
- ½ tsp chilli powder
- ¼ tsp salt
- 1 lb cooked chicken breast, shredded
- ½ cup part-skim mozzarella
- ½ cup low-fat Monterey Jack cheese, divided

DIRECTIONS

1. In a large bowl whisk together cream cheese, yogurt, enchilada sauce, green chillies, and spices.

2. Fold in the shredded chicken, mozzarella, and ¼ cup of cheese

3. Place all of the ingredients in the slow cooker and cook on low for 2 hours

4. Remove dip from the slow cooker and put it in a safe oven dish

5. Top with remaining cheese broiler until cheese is lightly browned

6. Serve with vegetables

NUTRITION FACTS: YIELD: 8 SERVING SIZE: 1

Amount Per Serving:

- CALORIES: 171

- TOTAL FAT: 7g

- SATURATED FAT: 4g

- TRANS FAT: 0g

- UNSATURATED FAT: 3g

- CHOLESTEROL: 50mg

- SODIUM: 415mg

- CARBOHYDRATES: 7g

- SUGAR: 4gPROTEIN: 19g

CHICKEN ENCHILADA SPAGHETTI SQUASH

YIELD: 4 servings

Per Serving: 1 Leaner, 3 Green, 1 Healthy Fat, 3 Condiment

INGREDIENTS

- 1 medium spaghetti squash
- 4 tsp olive oil, divided
- ½ tsp salt, divided
- ¼ tsp pepper
- 1 cup canned, diced tomatoes
- ½ cup chicken broth
- 1 Tbsp chilli powder
- ½ tsp cumin
- ½ tsp oregano
- ½ onion powder
- ½ jalapeno, stem and seeds removed
- 1 clove garlic
- 1 lb chicken breast, cooked and shredded
- 1 cup shredded, reduced fat cheddar Jack cheese
- ¼ cup cilantro, chopped

DIRECTIONS

1. Pre-set oven to 400°F

2. Prepare the spaghetti squash; cut in half and remove seed and pulp strands (two teaspoons total). Run one teaspoon olive oil into each squash half and season each with a quarter teaspoon salt and pepper. Place each spaghetti squash half faced down on a foil-lined baking sheet, and bake for 40-60 minutes, until the middle is tender and pulls apart easily

3. Meanwhile in a blender or food processor, combine tomatoes, chicken broth, chilli powder, cumin, oregano, onion powder, salt jalapeno, garlic, and the remaining 2 teaspoons of olive oil. Blend until smooth. Add sauce to the shredded chicken, mix until fully coated

4. When spaghetti squash is fully cooked, flip in the baking dish so that it is now skin-side down. Lightly scrape flesh with a fork to create spaghetti like strands.

5. Evenly divide chicken mixture between each squash half. Top each half with one-half cup of cheddar jack cheese, and sprinkle with cilantro

6. Turn oven to broil and cook for additional 3 to 5 minutes, until cheese is browned. Serve immediately.

NUTRITION FACTS

Serving Size:

- 1/2 Stuffed Squash Half Per Serving
- 408 calories; protein 34.3g;
- carbohydrates 19.7g;
- dietary fiber 4.1g;
- sugars 6.7g; fat 22.1g;
- saturated fat 11.1g;

- cholesterol 136.3mg;

- vitamin a iu 1113.1IU;

- vitamin c 19.3mg;

- folate 46.2mcg;

- calcium 278.5mg;

- iron 1.8mg;

- magnesium 71.5mg;

- potassium 832.9mg;

- sodium 425.9mg;

- thiamin 0.2mg.

- Exchanges: 1 Starch, 1 Vegetable, 3 1/2 Lean Meat, 1 High-Fat Meat

CHICKPEA & SWEET POTATO BREAKFAST HASH

Prep Time: 10 min

Cook Time: 40 min

Total Time: 50 minutes

Yield: Serves 3

INGREDIENTS

- 1 ½ lb. sweet potatoes, cut into ¾ – 1 inch cubes

- ½ large onion, chopped

- 1 red bell pepper, cored and diced

- 1 green bell pepper, cored and diced

- 1 can (15oz.) chickpeas (garbanzo beans), drained and rinsed

- 1 – 2 tablespoons olive oil

- 1 teaspoon garlic powder

- Generous pinch of mineral salt, or to taste

- Fresh cracked pepper, to taste

- Sriracha Tahini Sauce

- 4 tablespoons tahini

- 4 tablespoons water

- Juice of ½ small lemon

- Pinch of mineral salt

- Sriracha, to taste

INSTRUCTIONS

1. Preheat oven to 425 degrees F. Line a sheet pan with parchment paper, a Silpat, or lightly grease with oil.

2. Assemble: Place the sweet potatoes, onion, bell peppers and chickpeas on the center of the sheet pan, drizzle with olive oil, garlic powder, salt and pepper, toss well to coat. Arrange the sweet potato mixture in a single layer.

3. Roast 1: Place sheet pan in the oven, on the center rack, and cook for 20 minutes, stirring halfway through.

4. Roast 2: Turn heat up to 500 degrees F., stir a second time and continue baking for another 20 minutes, stirring halfway through. Let cool a few minutes.

5. Dressing: While the breakfast hash is roasting, whisk together the tahini, water, lemon, salt, and sriracha in a small bowl. Let rest for flavors to develop. Taste for flavor before serving.

NUTRITION FACTS:

- Calcium9%
- Iron15%
- Vitamin D0%
- Magnesium21%
- Potassium23%
- Zinc13%
- Phosphorus17%
- Thiamin (B1)21%
- Riboflavin (B2)17%
- Niacin (B3)14%
- Vitamin B650%
- Folic Acid (B9)25%
- Vitamin E14%
- Vitamin K14%

TEX-MEX TOFU BREAKFAST TACOS

- Servings: 4 (2 tacos per serving)
- Prep Time: 5 – 10 minutes
- Cooking Time: 15 minutes (Per Serving)
- Calories: 286

- Protein: 16 grams
- Carbohydrates: 26 grams
- Fat: 9 grams

INGREDIENTS

- 2 (14 ounce) packages soft tofu, drained
- 3 (6 inches) corn tortillas, cut into strips
- 1/8 teaspoon turmeric
- 1 jalapeño, seeded and diced
- 1/2 teaspoon smoked paprika
- 4 scallions, trimmed and chopped
- 1/2 teaspoon salt
- 1/4 cup fresh cilantro, chopped
- 2 plum tomatoes, diced
- 1/4 cup vegan cheese, shredded
- 8 (6 inches) corn tortillas, warmed
- 1/2 cup salsa (optional)

DIRECTIONS

1. Coat a large nonstick skillet in cooking spray and place over medium heat. Add the tortilla strips and sauté until golden and crispy, around 6 minutes. Transfer to a plate and set aside.

2. Recoat the pan in cooking spray. Add the tofu to the pan and crumble it into various-sized pieces similar to scrambled eggs. Add the turmeric, jalapeño,

paprika, scallions, and salt and stir until well combined.

3. Cook until the remaining water in the tofu has cooked off and it has a tender consistency, about 4 – 6 minutes. Add the cilantro, tomatoes, cheese, and tortilla strips. Stir until well combined. Continue stirring until cheese has melted, around 2 minutes.

4. Divide into 4 equal portions, then divide each portion between 2 corn tortillas. Top each taco with 1 tablespoon salsa

5. Serve and Enjoy!

MOCHA OATMEAL SERVINGS

Cooking Time: 5 minutes (Per Serving)

INGREDIENTS

- 1/2 cup old-fashioned oats
- 1/2 cup water
- 1/4 cup brewed coffee
- 1 tablespoon unsweetened cocoa powder
- 1 teaspoon stevia or another natural sweetener

DIRECTIONS

Cook oats according to package directions.

Mix in coffee, cocoa powder and stevia.

NUTRITIONAL FACTS:

- Servings Per Recipe: 1
- Amount Per Serving

- Calories: 158.2

- Total Fat: 3.4 g

- Cholesterol: 0.0 mg

- Sodium: 5.6 mg

- Total Carbs: 29.1 g

- Dietary Fiber: 4.9 g

- Protein: 5.8 g

PEANUT BUTTER & PROTEIN PANCAKES

Servings: 1

Prep Time: 5 mins

Cooking Time: 5 mins (Per Serving)

Calories: 397

Protein: 33 grams

Carbohydrates: 51 grams

Fat: 7 grams

INGREDIENTS

- 1/2 banana, mashed

- 2 teaspoons peanut butter

- 1 serving protein powder (of your choice)

- 1/3 cup whole grain pancake batter

- 1 teaspoon honey

DIRECTIONS

1. In a large mixing bowl, add the banana, peanut butter, protein powder, and batter and mix well

2. Coat a large nonstick skillet in cooking spray and place over medium heat. Divide the batter evenly in half and spoon onto the skillet.

3. Cook, turning when tops are covered with bubbles and edges look cooked.

4. Drizzle honey on top.

NUTRITION FACTS:

- Serving: 1pancake |
- Calories: 147kcal |
- Carbohydrates: 10g |
- Protein: 13g |
- Fat: 7g |
- SaturatedFat: 2g |
- Cholesterol: 44mg |
- Sodium: 265mg |
- Potassium: 192mg |
- Fiber: 2g |
- Sugar: 4g |
- Vitamin A: 79IU |
- Vitamin C: 2mg |
- Calcium: 156mg |
- Iron: 1mg

CAPRESE CHICKEN

YIELD: 4 Servings

Per Serving: 1 Leaner, 3 Green, 3 Condiment, 1 Healthy Fat

Total Time: 30 Minutes

INGREDIENTS:

- 2 tsp olive oil
- 2 garlic cloves, minced
- 1 cups grape tomatoes, halved
- 3 Tbsp balsamic vinegar
- ¼ tsp each salt and pepper
- ½ cup fresh basil leaves, torn into pieces
- 4.4oz boneless and skinless chicken breast butterflies then pounded very thin (⅛ -¼ inches thick)
- 2 cup reduced-fat shredded mozzarella

DIRECTIONS

1. Heat olive oil in a large skillet over medium-high heat. Add garlic, and stir for one minute. Add tomatoes, balsamic vinegar, salt and pepper. Cover and cook for 8 to 10 minutes, until tomatoes have softened. Remove from heat and stir in fresh basil. Grill or sauté chicken breast over medium-high heat for few minutes on each side until fully cooked

2. Transfer to a baking sheet. Top chicken with tomato mixture and mozzarella cheese, as if it were a pizza.

3. Broil for 2 to 5 minutes or until cheese is melted.

Tip: Serve with a vegetable such as broccoli or asparagus (1 cup of either option per serving) to make a complete lean or green meal.

NUTRITION FACTS

- Calories from Fat 92
- Calories 247% Daily Value*15%
- Total Fat 10g
- Saturated Fat 3.4g
- *Trans* Fat 0g
- Polyunsaturated Fat 1.3g
- Grams Monounsaturated Fat 4.7g; Cholesterol 98mg
- Sodium 461mg
- Potassium 325mg
- Total Carbohydrates 1.5g
- Dietary Fiber 0.4g
- Sugars 0.8g
- Protein 35g.

INSTANT POT MOROCCAN CHICKEN

YIELD: 4 Servings

Per Serving: 1 Leaner, 3 Green, 2½ Condiment, 1 Healthy Fat

Total Time: 30 Minutes

INGREDIENTS

- 1 tsp nutmeg
- 1 tsp cumin
- 1 tsp coriander
- ½ tsp allspice
- ½ ground ginger
- ⅛ tsp cayenne
- ⅛ tsp cinnamon
- ½ tsp salt
- ½ tsp pepper
- 2 pounds boneless skinless chicken breast, cubed
- 2 diced tomatoes
- ½ cup chicken broth
- 20 green, pitted olives
- ½ Tbsp olive oil
- 4 cups frozen rice cauliflower

DIRECTIONS

- Combine the first nine ingredients in a large, re-sealable plastic bag. Add chicken, and toss to coat.
- Place chicken in Instant Pot, and top with canned tomatoes and juices, chicken broth, olives and olive oil. Secure lid and close pressure valve. Set to 20 minutes at high pressure. Allow pressure to release naturally before opening.

- Meanwhile, microwave or sauté (using little cooking spray) riced cauliflower according to package directions.
- Serve chicken and sauce atop cauliflower rice.

NUTRITION FACTS

- Serving Size:
- 1/6 Calories: 346
- Sugar: 7 Fat: 15
- Carbohydrates: 30
- Fiber: 4 Protein: 26

HEALTHY FRENCH TOAST SERVINGS

Prep Time: 2 minutes

Cooking Time: 5 minutes (Per Serving)

Calories: 421

INGREDIENTS

- 14 egg whites
- 1/4 cup skim milk
- 1/8 teaspoon cinnamon
- 1/2 scoop vanilla whey protein powder
- 2 slices whole grain bread
- 1 banana, sliced or 1 1/2 cups mixed berries

DIRECTIONS

1. In a medium-sized mixing bowl, add the egg whites, milk, cinnamon, and protein powder and whisk until thoroughly combined.

2. Coat a large nonstick skillet in cooking spray and place over medium heat. 3. Soak the bread in the egg white mixture for 10 – 15 seconds, then place it in the skillet. Cook for 2 – 3 minutes, then flip.

3. Pour the egg mixture into the pan around the bread and cook.

4. Transfer to a plate then top with banana or berries.

NUTRITION FACT:

- Protein: 38 grams

- Carbohydrates: 60 grams

- Fat: 4 grams

- Vitamin B-12 (41.25%)

- Vitamin B6 (22.54%)

- Sodium (19.47%)

- Selenium (18.00%)

- Vitamin B2 (17.31%)

ORANGE RICOTTA PANCAKES

Servings:6 (2 pancakes per serving)

Prep Time: 5 mins

Cooking Time: 10 mins (Per Serving)

Calories: 242

Protein: 21 grams

Carbohydrates: 27 grams

Fat: 5 grams

INGREDIENTS

- 1 cup barley flour
- 1/3 cup all-purpose flour
- 2 tablespoons stevia or another natural sweetener
- 3 scoops vanilla whey protein powder
- 2 teaspoons baking powder
- 1/2 teaspoon baking soda
- 1 cup fat free ricotta cheese
- 1/2 cup skim milk
- 1/2 cup orange juice
- 1 teaspoon orange zest
- 2 large eggs, beaten
- 1 tablespoon unsalted butter
- 1 teaspoon vanilla extract

DIRECTIONS

1. In a large mixing bowl, add the barley, flour, stevia, protein powder, baking powder, and baking soda and mix until well combined. Set aside.

2. In a separate large mixing bowl, add the ricotta, skim milk, orange juice, orange zest, eggs, butter, and vanilla extract. Beat together until mixed well. Slowly

mix liquid ingredients into dry ingredients until just mixed. Do not over-mix.

3. Coat a large nonstick skillet in cooking spray and wipe away the excess with a paper towel. Save this for wiping the pan after each pancake. Heat the skillet over medium heat.

4. Spoon about 3 to 4 tablespoons of batter onto the griddle and cook until bubbles appear. Flip and cook until golden brown. 5. Repeat step 4 with the remaining batter.

NUTRITION FACTS:

- Per Serving: 527 calories;

- total fat 9g; saturated fat 5g;

- polyunsaturated fat 1g;

- monounsaturated fat 3g;

- cholesterol 97mg; sodium 551mg;

- potassium 348mg; carbohydrates 99g; fiber 5g; sugar 54g; protein 13g; trans fatty acid 0g;

OATMEAL CEREAL SERVINGS

- Prep Time: 3 – 4 mins (Per Serving)

- Calories: 496

- Protein: 30 grams

- Carbohydrates: 47 grams

- Fat: 23 grams

INGREDIENTS

1. 1/2 cup old-fashioned oats
2. 1/2 scoop vanilla whey protein powder
3. 1/4 teaspoon cinnamon
4. 1/4 teaspoon stevia or another natural sweetener
5. 1/8 teaspoon vanilla extract
6. Salt, to taste
7. 2 tablespoons almond butter
8. 1 cup skim milk

DIRECTIONS

1. In a medium-sized bowl, add the oats, protein powder, cinnamon, stevia, vanilla extract, and salt. Mix together well.
2. Add the almond butter, one small chunk at a time. Stir into the mixture allowing it to break up slightly until it resembles crumbly cookie dough.
3. Top with skim milk.

NUTRITION FACTS

- Fat: 23 g.
- Saturated Fat: 0.5 g.
- Cholesterol: 0 mg.
- Protein: 30 g.
- Carbohydrates: 47 g.
- Sugar: 15 g.

CHEESY CHICKEN CAULIFLOWER SKILLET

YIELD: 4 Servings

Per Serving: 1 Lean, 3 Green, 1 Condiment

Time: 20 minutes

INGREDIENTS

- 1½ cup (4 oz) sliced mushrooms
- 1.12-oz bag frozen riced cauliflower
- 2 cloves garlic, minced
- 2 tsp olive oil
- ½ cup chicken broth
- 1.12-oz can be shredded chicken breast, drained
- 8 oz reduced fat shredded mozzarella cheese
- ½ tsp dried oregano
- 2 scallions chopped

DIRECTIONS

1. Cook mushrooms, cauliflower, and garlic in oil for 3 to 4 minutes. Pour in broth, and bring to a boil.

2. Add chicken, reduce heat, and simmer 4 to 5 minutes or until vegetables are tender and chicken is heated through. Stir in mozzarella and oregano; top with scallions.

NUTRITION FACT:

- Serving: 11/2 cups,

- Calories: 263kcal, Carbohydrates: 11g,

- Protein: 35g, Fat: 9g, Saturated Fat: 3g,

- Cholesterol: 96mg, Sodium: 485mg,

- Fiber: 4g, Sugar: 3.5g

CHICKEN ENCHILADA ROLL UPS

YIELD: 4 Servings

Per Serving: 1 Leaner, 1 Healthy Fat, 3 Green, 1½ Condiments

Total Time: 45-50 Minutes

INGREDIENTS

- 1 tsp cumin

- 1 tsp dried oregano

- 1 tsp garlic powder

- 1 tsp chilli powder

- 1.10oz can mild red enchilada sauce

- 1.14oz can mild green chillies

- ½ cup diced tomatoes

- 4.6oz raw boneless skinless chicken breast, butterflied

- 1 cup reduced-fat shredded Mexican cheese blend, divided

- 3 cups grated cauliflower

- 1.4½-oz avocado, cubed

- ¼ cup chopped cilantro (optional)

DIRECTIONS

1. Pre- heat oven to 375°F

2. In a small bowl, combine the cumin, oregano, garlic powder, chilli powder. Rub in both sides of each chicken piece

3. In a lightly greased baking dish, pour a thin layer of enchilada sauce on the bottom of the dish.

4. Lay chicken, cut side up on a work surface. Top each piece, in the center, with about 2 teaspoons chillies, 1 tablespoon chopped tomatoes, and 2 tablespoons cheese. Roll each one up and set them seam side down the baking dish. Top with the remaining sauce, chillies, tomatoes and cheese.

5. Cover with foil and bake for 30 minutes. Remove foil and continue to bake 10 to 15 minutes more, or until chicken is cooked through.

6. Meanwhile, microwave grated cauliflower with 1 tablespoon water in the microwave 6 to 8 minutes or until tender.

7. Place each chicken roll-up on a bed of cauliflower rice, and top with avocado and fresh cilantro.

NUTRITION FACT:

- Serving: 1roll-upwith1ounce
  avocado, Calories: 261kcal, Carbohydrates: 8g,

- Protein: 31g, Fat: 11.5g,

- Saturated

  Fat: 3.5g, Cholesterol: 83mg, Sodium: 658mg, Fiber: 3g, Sugar: 1g

BLACK BEAN + SWEET POTATO HASH (OIL FREE)

Serves: 4

Time: About 15 minutes (5 minutes prep time, 10 minutes cook time)

Total calories: 133

Protein: 5

Carbs: 28

Fiber: 9.5

Fat: 1

INGREDIENTS

- 2 cups peeled, chopped sweet potatoes
- 1 cup chopped onion
- 1 cup cooked and drained black beans
- 1 minced garlic clove
- ⅓ cup veggie broth
- ¼ cup chopped scallions
- 2 teaspoons hot chili powder

DIRECTIONS

1. Prep your veggies.

2. Turn your pressure cooker to "sauté" and cook the chopped onion for 2-3 minutes, stirring so it doesn't burn.

3. Add the garlic and stir until fragrant.

4. Add the sweet potatoes and chili powder, and stir.

5. Pour in the broth and give one last stir before locking the lid.

6. Select "manual," and cook on high pressure for 3 minutes.

7. When time is up, quick-release the pressure carefully.

8. Add the black beans and scallions, and stir to heat everything.

9. Season with salt and more chili powder if desired.

NUTRITION FACTS:

- Serving Size (1/3 of recipe):
- Calories 255 Total Fat 10g
- Saturated Fat 1g Sodium 285mg
- Total Carbohydrates 33g Fiber 9g Protein 11g

CRANBERRY-WALNUT QUINOA (OIL FREE)

Serves: 4

Time: 10 minutes

Total calories: 611

Protein: 13

Carbs: 85

Fiber: 5.25

Fat: 1

INGREDIENTS

- 2 cups water
- 2 cups dried cranberries
- 1 cup quinoa
- 1 cup chopped walnuts
- 1 cup sunflower seeds
- ½ tablespoon cinnamon

DIRECTIONS

1. Rinse quinoa
2. Put quinoa, water, and salt in the pressure cooker
3. Lock the lid.
4. Select "manual," and cook for 10 minutes on high pressure.
5. When the timer beeps, hit "cancel" and quick-release.
6. When the pressure is gone, open the cooker
7. Mix in the dried cranberries, nuts, seeds, sweetener, and cinnamon
8. Serve and enjoy!

NUTRITION FACTS

- Amount per serving
- calories 157

- calories from fat 54

Fat 6g 9% sodium 248mg 11% potassium 190mg 5% carbohydrates 21g 7% fiber 2g 8% sugar 1g 1% protein 4g 8% vitamin a 170iu 3% vitamin c 10.6mg 13% calcium 17mg 2% iron 1.4mg 8%

EGGS & QUINOA INSTANT BREAKFAST

- Servings: 1 Prep
- Time: 1 min
- Cooking Time: Under 5 mins (Per Serving)
- Calories: 286
- Protein: 22 grams
- Carbohydrates: 40 grams
- Fat: 5 grams

INGREDIENTS

- 4 egg whites
- 2/3 cup quinoa, cooked 1/3 cup almond milk
- 1 teaspoon maple syrup
- 1/2 cup mixed berries

DIRECTIONS

1. Add the egg whites to a microwave-safe bowl. Cover with paper towel or lid and microwave for 2 – 3 minutes or until cooked.

2. Add quinoa and almond milk to the bowl.

3. Microwave for 1 minute.

4. Top with maple syrup and berries.

VEGAN BLUEBERRY BANANA OAT BREAD

This vegan blueberry banana bread is moist, super easy to make and not overly sweet. Plus, it's made with heart healthy, wholesome ingredients.

Prep Time: 15 min Cook Time: 50 min

Yield: Makes 8 - 10 slices

Category: Quick Bread

Cuisine: Vegan

INGREDIENTS

- 1 ¼ cups (120g) old fashioned oats
- 1 ¼ cups (125g) light spelled flour
- ⅓ cup (47g) sugar (turbinado, coconut or pure cane)
- 2 teaspoons baking powder
- ½ teaspoon baking soda
- Generous pinch of salt
- 2 – 3 ripe bananas, mashed (about 1 to 1 ¼ cups (220-276g))
- ¼ cup (56ml) unsweetened almond milk
- ¼ cup (56ml) grapeseed or light flavored olive oil or applesauce
- 1 cup (100g) fresh blueberries (frozen is ok too)

- optional add ins

- 1 teaspoon vanilla extract

- 1 teaspoon cinnamon

INSTRUCTIONS

1. Preheat oven to 350 degrees F.

2. Grease a 9 x 5 loaf pan lightly with oil.

3. Combine: In a medium sized mixing bowl, add the flour, oats, sugar, baking powder, baking soda, optional cinnamon and a pinch of salt, stir to combine.

4. Mash the bananas by hand in a small bowl, using the back of a fork or slotted spoon.

5. Mix: To the dry ingredients, add the mashed bananas, oil, plant milk and optional vanilla, mix to combine, just until the flour is incorporated. Best practice for mixing quick bread batter: Don't overmix, as overmixing the ingredients will cause the gluten proteins to create an elastic batter that will not rise well.

6. Gently fold in the blueberries.

7. Pour the batter into a lightly greased 9 x 5 loaf pan. Optionally, add a few blueberries strategically to the top and sprinkle a small handful of oats over the top. I added quick oats, but old fashioned oat would look nice too. You can also chop old fashioned oats into smaller pieces.

8. Bake: Place loaf pan in the oven and bake for 50 – 55 minutes, rotating the pan once halfway through. The top will turn golden and the toothpick placed in the center will come out clean.

9. Once done, let cool for 15 minutes in the pan. You should tilt the pan and the loaf will come out clean, place on a rack to cool completely.

NUTRITION FACTS:

- Serving: 1slice | Calories: 153kcal | Carbohydrates: 21 g |

- Protein: 2g | Fat: 6g | Sodium: 195mg | Potassium: 94 mg | Fiber: 1g |

- Vitamin A: 372IU Vitamin C: 2mg Calcium: 10mg Iron: 1mg NET CARBS: 20g

HEALTHY HOMEMADE GRANOLA RECIPE (OIL-FREE)

Naturally sweetened with maple syrup and oil-free, this delicious crunchy granola is versatile and perfect at any time of day!

Prep Time: 10 min Cook Time: 45 min

Yield: 6 cups (12 servings)

Category: Breakfast, Snack

Cuisine: Vegan

INGREDIENTS

- 3 cups old fashioned oats
- 1 cup raw almonds, whole or slivered
- 1 cup raw cashews, whole or halves & pieces
- 1 cup coconut flakes or shredded coconut
- ¼ cup flaxseed meal

- ½ cup pure maple syrup

- 1 tablespoon vanilla extract

- ½ teaspoon cinnamon, optional

- Pinch of salt

INSTRUCTIONS

1. Prep: Preheat oven to 300 degrees Fahrenheit. Line large, rimmed baking sheet with parchment paper or a Silpat.

2. Combine: In a large mixing bowl, combine the oats, almonds, cashews, flaxseed meal, coconut flakes, maple syrup, vanilla, optional cinnamon and a pinch of salt, mix well to combine.

3. Spread: Layer granola mixture on the lined baking sheet, spreading out to the edges, as evenly distributed as possible.

4. Bake: Place baking sheet in the oven, on the middle rack, and cook for 45 minutes, stirring the mixture well every 10 minutes or so.

5. Let cool slightly: Once done, remove from oven and let cool. When the granola has cooled, it will be perfectly crunchy and ready for you to devour!

6. Store: Keep leftover granola in an air tight container for up to 3 weeks.

7. Makes 6 cups, with 12 servings

8. Ways to serve your granola:

9. It's great as a cereal with fresh fruit, non-dairy milk or yogurt.

10. Topped on non-dairy ice cream

11. Add a small handful on top of your favorite smoothies, smoothie bowls and shakes

12. Add in ½ – 1 cup of dried fruit once the granola has been pulled from the oven. A few dried fruits to use are raisins, dried blueberries or cranberries.

NUTRITION FACTS

- **Serving Size:** 1/10 of the recipe

- **Calories:** 262

- **Sugar:** 29g

- **Sodium:** 4mg

- **Fat:** 7.5g

- **Saturated Fat:** 0.7g

- **Carbohydrates:** 46.8g

- **Fiber:** 5.5g

- **Protein:** 5.3g

CHOCOLATE ALMOND BUTTER SMOOTHIE BOWL

Whip up a bowl of pure bliss with this dreamy and creamy chocolate almond butter smoothie bowl. Easy to make and refined sugar-free. Makes a great treat any time of day!

Prep Time: 5 min Total Time: 5 minutes

- Yield: Serves 2

- Category: Smoothie, Breakfast

- Method: blender

- Cuisine: Vegan

- 2 large frozen bananas (pref. overripe)
- ¼ cup almond butter (or your favorite nut butter)
- 2 tablespoons cocoa powder
- 1 teaspoon vanilla extract, optional
- 1 cup unsweetened almond milk
- 3 – 4 ice cubes
- Optional toppings
- Sliced bananas
- Granola
- Cocoa nibs
- Chopped almonds

INSTRUCTIONS

Place bananas, almond butter, cocoa powder, optional vanilla, milk and ice cubes into the blender, blend until smooth. Serve in small to medium-sized bowls with optional toppings of choice. For a more traditional smoothie, serve in a glass with a few of the optional toppings. Use a wide straw or spoon.

NOTES

Add a level scoop of protein powder for extra protein. Use a tad more milk as needed, a splash or two at a time.

If you don't mind a little added sugar, try Silk's Protein & Nut Milk with this recipe. It contains 10 grams of protein per and 2 grams of sugar per serving.

BANANA-BUCKWHEAT PORRIDGE (OIL FREE)

Serves: 3-4

Time: 26 minutes (6 minutes cook time, 20 minutes natural release)

Total calories: 240

Protein: 6

Carbs: 46

Fiber: 5

Fat: 4

Buckwheat is a good oat alternative if you're sensitive to gluten. It's also high in fiber and has comparable health benefits to fruits and veggies! Because of its texture, buckwheat takes a little longer to cook than rolled oats, so you need to do a natural pressure release to make sure it's soft enough.

INGREDIENTS

- 3 cups almond (or rice) milk
- 1 cup buckwheat groats
- 1 sliced banana
- ¼ cup raisins
- 1 teaspoon cinnamon
- ½ teaspoon pure vanilla extract

DIRECTIONS

1. Rinse off the buckwheat and put it right in the pressure cooker

2. Pour in the milk, and add the rest of the ingredients

3. Lock the lid

4. Select "manual," and then cook for 6 minutes on high pressure.

5. When time is up, hit "cancel" and wait 20 minutes or so for the pressure to go all the way down.

6. Open the lid and stir well. Add more milk if it's too thick for you.

7. Serve!

NUTRITIONAL FACTS:

YIELD: 8   SERVING SIZE: 1

- *Amount per serving:* calories: 155 total fat: 8g

- Saturated   fat: 1gtrans   fat: 0g;   unsaturated fat: 6gcholesterol: 0mg

- Sodium: 137mg;   carbohydrates: 18g;   fiber: 4g; sugar: 5g; protein: 6g

PEAR OATS WITH WALNUTS

Serves: - 4

Time: 6 minutes

Total calories: 288

Protein: 5

Carbs: 39

Fiber: 4.5

Fat: 13

Rolled oats are one of the fastest cooking foods with the pressure cooker. You mix everything in a bowl for this recipe, which sets in the steamer rack in the cooker. The oats cook in almond milk, sugar, and just a tablespoon of coconut oil. Fresh pears will soften beautifully in there, as well, and you finish it off with cinnamon and walnuts.

INGREDIENTS:

- 2 cups almond milk

- 2 cups peeled and cut pears

- 1 cup rolled oats

- ½ cup chopped walnuts

- ¼ cup sugar

- 1 tablespoon melted coconut oil

- ¼ teaspoon salt Dash of cinnamon

DIRECTIONS:

1. Mix everything except the walnuts and cinnamon in an oven-safe bowl that you know fits in the pressure cooker.

2. Pour 1 cup of water into the pressure cooker and lower it in a steamer rack.

3. Put the bowl on top and lock the lid.

4. Select "manual," and then high pressure for 6 minutes.

5. When time is up, quick-release the pressure.

6. Carefully remove the bowl, divide into 4 servings, and season with salt and cinnamon.

NUTRITION FACTS:

YIELD: 8 Serving Size: 1

- *Amount Per Serving:* Calories: 203total
- Fat: 8g
- saturated Fat: 2g
- trans Fat: 0g
- unsaturated Fat: 6g
- cholesterol: 27mg
- sodium: 169mg
- Carbohydrates: 28g; fiber: 5g; sugar: 7g; protein: 7g

SPICY TEX-MEX BREAKFAST BURRITO

Servings: 1

Prep Time: 5 mins

Cooking Time: 5 mins (Per Serving)

Calories: 294

Protein: 28 grams

Carbohydrates: 42 grams

Fat: 5 grams

INGREDIENTS

- 1 (10 inches) whole grain tortilla
- 1/2 teaspoon jalapeño, seeded and diced
- 2 tablespoons red bell pepper, diced

- 2 tablespoons green bell pepper, diced
- 2 tablespoons onion, diced
- 2 tablespoons tomato, diced
- 5 egg whites
- 1 tablespoon low-fat cheddar cheese, shredded
- 1 tablespoon fresh cilantro, chopped

DIRECTIONS

1. Coat a medium-sized skillet in cooking spray and place over medium heat.

2. Add the jalapeños, bell peppers, onion, and tomato. Sauté for 2 – 3 minutes, or until tender.

3. Pour in the eggs and scramble. Once cooked, transfer the egg mixture to a plate.

4. Place the tortilla in the hot pan and warm, about 1 minute on each side. Remove tortilla from heat and top with egg mixture, sprinkle with cheese and cilantro.

5. Serve!

NUTRITIONAL FACTS:

YIELD: 4 SERVING SIZE: 1 burrito

Amount Per Serving: CALORIES: 1107; TOTAL FAT: 58g

SATURATED FAT: 22g TRANS FAT: 1g

UNSATURATED FAT: 30g CHOLESTEROL: 498mg

SODIUM: 2597mg

CARBOHYDRATES: 86g FIBER: 13g SUGAR: 7g

PROTEIN: 61g

BREAKFAST TOFU SCRAMBLE (OIL FREE)

Serves: 4

Time: 9 minutes (5 minutes prep time, 4 minutes cook time)

Total calories: 139

Protein: 12

Carbs: 15

Fiber: 1

Fat: 5

Breakfast scrambles are quick, easy, and you can add just about anything you want. This recipe includes cherry tomatoes, a potato, and an apple. Instead of eggs, you use crumbled tofu. Seasonings are up to you, as well, and since tofu is pretty bland, don't be shy.

INGREDIENTS:

- 1 block of extra-firm, crumbled tofu
- 1 cup cherry tomatoes
- 1 onion
- 1 diced potato
- 1 diced apple
- ¼ cup veggie broth
- 2 minced garlic cloves
- 1 teaspoon dry dill ½ teaspoon ground turmeric.

- Salt and pepper to taste

DIRECTIONS:

1. Turn your pressure cooker to sauté and dry-cook the garlic and onion until the onion begins to soften

2. Add a bit of water if it starts to stick.

3. Pour broth into the cooker, and add the rest of the ingredients.

4. Select "manual" and cook on high pressure for 4 minutes.

5. When time is up, hit "cancel" and quick-release.

6. Stir, season to taste, and enjoy!

NUTRITION FACTS

Calories: 224kcal | Carbohydrates: 15g |

Protein: 22g | Fat: 9g | SaturatedFat: 1g | Sodium: 69mg | Potassium: 446mg | Fiber: 6g | Sugar: 4g | Vitamin A: 1660IU | Vitamin C: 80mg | Calcium: 255mg | Iron: 3mg

PUMPKIN SPICE OATMEAL WITH BROWN SUGAR TOPPING (OIL FREE)

Serves: 6-8

Time: 15 minutes (3 minutes cook time, 12 minutes natural release)

Total calories: 207

Protein: 4

Carbs: 38

Fiber: 4

Fat: 4

If someone tells you that vegan food is bland, serve them this breakfast and they'll change their mind. It uses steel-cut oats, pumpkin puree, cinnamon, and allspice. The brown sugar, chopped pecan topping is just as delicious and adds a nice crunch. Cooking Tip: If you like really soft oats, cook for at least 7 minutes instead of 3.

INGREDIENTS:

- 4 ½ cups water
- 1 ½ cups steel-cut oats
- 1 ½ cups pumpkin puree
- 2 teaspoons cinnamon
- 1 teaspoon vanilla
- 1 teaspoon allspice
- ½ cup brown sugar
- ¼ cup chopped pecans
- 1 tablespoon cinnamon

DIRECTIONS:

1. Pour 1 cup of water into the pressure cooker
2. Add everything from the first ingredient list (including the rest of the water) into an oven-safe bowl and set it in the steamer basket.
3. Lower the basket into the pressure cooker and lock the lid.
4. Select "manual," and cook on high pressure for 3 minutes.

5. When time is up, hit "cancel" and wait for the pressure to come down on its own.

6. Mix the topping ingredients in a small bowl.

7. When you serve, sprinkle on top. If necessary, add a little almond milk to the oats.

NUTRITION FACTS:

Calories: 345kcal | Carbohydrates: 51g | Protein: 9g | Fat: 13 g | Saturated
Fat: 4g | Cholesterol: 60mg | Sodium: 337mg | Potassium: 3 98mg | Fiber: 6g | Sugar: 27g | Vitamin A: 6529IU | Vitamin C: 3mg | Calcium: 118mg | Iron: 2mg

COCONUT-ALMOND RISOTTO (OIL FREE)

Serves: 4

Time: 20 minutes (10 minutes cook time, 10 minutes natural release)

Risotto is usually reserved for savory side dishes, but it's a perfect vehicle for sweeter breakfasts, too. Using vanilla almond milk and coconut milk adds flavor and a beautiful creaminess. For texture, a topping of coconut flakes and sliced almonds is perfect.

Total calories: 337

Protein: 6

Carbs: 66

Fiber: 1.5

Fat: 7

INGREDIENTS:

- 2 cups vanilla almond milk
- 1 cup coconut milk
- 1 cup Arborio rice
- ⅓ cup sugar
- 2 teaspoons pure vanilla
- ¼ cup sliced almonds and coconut flakes

DIRECTIONS:

1. Pour the milk into the pressure cooker and hit the "sauté" button.
2. Stir until it boils.
3. Add the rice and stir before locking the lid.
4. Select "manual," and cook for 5 minutes on high pressure.
5. When time is up, press "cancel" and waits 10 minutes. Quick-release any leftover pressure.
6. Add the sugar and vanilla.
7. Divide up oats and top with almonds and coconut.
8. Enjoy!

NUTRITION FACTS:

- Saturated Fat 22g Trans Fat 0g Unsaturated Fat7g
- **Cholesterol** 0mg **Sodium**307 mg
- **Carbohydrates**25g Fiber2g Sugar5g **Protein**7g

PROTEIN OATCAKES

Servings: 2 (2 pancakes per serving)

Prep Time: 3 mins

Cooking Time: 5 – 6 mins (Per Serving)

Calories: 223

Protein: 31 grams

Carbohydrates: 20 grams

Fat: 2 grams

INGREDIENTS

- 1/2 cup old-fashioned oats
- 1/2 cup fat-free cottage cheese
- 6 egg whites • 1/2 teaspoon cinnamon
- 1/2 teaspoon vanilla extract
- 1/8 teaspoon baking powder
- 1 scoop vanilla whey protein powder

DIRECTIONS

1. Place all ingredients in a large mixing bowl and mix with a whisk or electric hand mixer until it thickens into a batter.

2. Coat a large nonstick skillet in cooking spray and wipe away the excess with a paper towel. Save this for wiping the pan after cooking each pancake. Heat the skillet over medium heat.

3. Pour or ladle about 1/2 cup of the batter onto the skillet and cook, 2 – 3 minutes for each side until golden brown. Repeat for the remaining batter.

4. Serve and Enjoy!

NUTRITION FACT:

- Calories 385.8 Total Fat   9.4 g Saturated Fat   3.3   g Polyunsaturated Fat2.9 g Monounsaturated Fat3.8 g

- Cholesterol   173.2 mg Sodium   349.7mg Potassium613.6 mg

- Total Carbohydrate 67.6 g Dietary Fiber 8.6g Sugars12.9 g Protein23.8 g

- Folate 19.9 % Iron   27.0 % Magnesium 38.5% Manganese   214.2 %

- Niacin 4.6 % Pantothenic Acid   15.6% Phosphorus64.8 % Riboflavin   28.1 %

- Selenium 10.3 % Thiamin   42.6 % Zinc 32.7 %

SUPER BERRY ACAI BOWL

Rich in antioxidants, vitamins, and minerals, this quick and easy homemade acai bowl is a perfect way to lighten up and cool down!

Prep Time: 5 min

Yield: Serves 1

Category: Breakfast, Smoothie

INGREDIENTS

- 1 cup frozen berry mix (any combo: blackberries, blueberries, strawberries, raspberries)

- 1 large banana (sliced and frozen)

- 1 tablespoon acai berry powder or 1 packet of frozen acai puree
- 1 cup unsweetened non-dairy milk or water, + more as needed
- 1 tablespoon nut butter, optional for protein
- Topping
- Mix of fresh berries and fruit
- Granola
- Toasted coconut flakes
- Chia seeds and/or hemp hearts

INSTRUCTIONS

1. In a blender, place the berries, banana, acai powder, optional protein source and water/milk. Blend until smooth. Add extra water if needed (most likely you won't need any).

2. Place in serving bowl and top with the suggested toppings or your favorite assortment.

3. Serves 1 large bowl or 2 small

NOTES

We recommend this acai berry powder from Terrasoul, purchased from Amazon. You can find frozen acai berry packets for smoothie bowls at Target in the freezer section with the other frozen fruits.

NUTRITIONAL FACTS

- Serving Size 173.00 g Servings Per Container

- Calories 230 Total Fat 6g9% Saturated Fat 2g10% Trans Fat 0g Cholesterol 0mg0%

- Sodium 30mg1% Total Carbohydrate 48g16% Dietary Fiber 4g16% Sugars 16g

- Protein 3g

CHAI-SPICED OATMEAL WITH MANGO (OIL FREE)

- Serves: 2-3 Time: 13 minutes (3 minutes cook time, 10 minutes natural release) A fan of chai tea?

- Total calories: 271

- Protein: 8

- Carbs: 47

- Fiber: 3.25

- Fat: 6

This oatmeal mimics those spicy-sweet flavors with cinnamon, ginger, cloves, and cardamom. The measurements are in "dashes," because it's up to you how much of each spice you want, depending on your tastes. Top the bowl off with some fresh-cut mango, or whatever fruit you like.

Cooking Tip: Cardamom and cloves are really strong, so add a teeny amount and taste.

INGREDIENTS

- 3 cups water

- 1 cup steel-cut oats

- ½ teaspoon vanilla

- Dash of cinnamon

- Dash of ginger

- Dash of cloves

- Dash of cardamom

- Dash of salt ½ mango, cut into pieces

DIRECTIONS

- Mix water and oats in the pressure cooker.

- Close the lid.

- Select "manual," and cook for 3 minutes on high pressure.

- When the beeper sounds, hit "cancel" and wait for the pressure to come down naturally.

- Open the lid and stir well.

- Season and taste.

- Divide into even servings and add chopped mango.

NUTRITIONAL FACTS:

- Total Fat 6.9g 9%

- Saturated Fat 1g

- Polyunsaturated Fat 2.9g

- Monounsaturated Fat 2.6g 0%

- Cholesterol 9.2mg   3%

- Sodium 104.7mg   5%

- Total Carbohydrate 19.4g   7%

- Dietary Fiber 2.1g   8%

- Sugars 7.2g

- Protein 4.3g 9%

BANANA-AMARANTH PORRIDGE (OIL FREE)

Serves: 4

Time: 13 minutes (3 minutes cook time, 10 minutes natural release)

Amaranth is an ancient "grain," though it technically isn't a grain at all. It's basically a bud, but has similar health benefits to other cereals, and it makes a darn tasty hot porridge. This recipe uses no added sugar; bananas add sweetness.

INGREDIENTS

- 2 ½ cups unsweetened almond milk

- 1 cup amaranth

- 2 sliced bananas

- Dash of cinnamon

DIRECTIONS

1. Mix the amaranth, milk, and bananas in your pressure cooker.

2. Seal the lid.

3. Select "manual," and cook on high pressure for just 3 minutes.

4. When time is up, hit "cancel" and wait for the pressure to come down on its own.

5. When all the pressure is gone, you can serve the porridge with cinnamon.

NUTRITIONAL FACTS:

- Total Fat 10g15% Saturated Fat 1g5% Trans Fat g Cholesterol 0mg0%

- Sodium 80mg3% Potassium 300mg9% Total Carbohydrates 22g7% Dietary Fiber 3g12%

- Sugars 14g Protein 2g4% Vitamin A4% Vitamin C10% Calcium4% Iron4%

LUNCH AND MAIN RECIPES

SPINACH AND TOFU SCRAMBLE

Servings: 2 Prep Time: Under 5 minutes

INGREDIENTS

- 2 tomatoes, diced
- 2 cloves garlic, minced
- 3/4 cup fresh mushrooms, sliced
- 1 cup spinach, rinsed
- 2 1/2 cups firm or extra firm tofu, crumbled
- 1/2 teaspoon low-sodium soy sauce
- 1 teaspoon lemon juice
- Salt and ground black pepper, to taste

DIRECTIONS

1. Coat a medium-sized skillet in cooking spray and place over medium heat.

2. Add the tomatoes, garlic, and mushrooms and sauté for 2 – 3 minutes.

3. Reduce heat to medium-low and add the spinach, tofu, soy sauce, and lemon juice. Cover with a tight fitting lid and cook for 5 – 7 minutes, stirring occasionally.

4. Sprinkle with salt and pepper.

NUTRITION FACTS:

1. Calories 284.4 Total Fat 14.3 g Saturated Fat3.0 g

2. Polyunsaturated Fat0.6 g Monounsaturated Fat3.3 g

3. Cholesterol 0.0 mg Sodium 991.9 mg Potassium 642.6 mg

4. Total Carbohydrate 14.4 g Dietary Fiber 6.0   g Sugars1.5 g Protein 25.4 g

TEMPEH HASH

Servings: 4

Prep Time: 5 minutes

Cooking Time: 25 minutes (Per Serving)

INGREDIENTS

- 12 ounces tempeh, cut into 1/2-inch cubes

- 4 medium potatoes, peeled and diced

- 1 onion, diced

- 2 tablespoons low-sodium soy sauce

- 1/2 teaspoon garlic powder

- Salt and ground black pepper, to taste

DIRECTIONS

1. Place the potatoes in a large pot, add water until the potatoes are just covered. Bring to a boil over medium-high heat and cook for 10 – 15 minutes, or until tender.

2. Coat a large skillet in cooking spray and place over medium heat. Add the onions, potatoes, tempeh, and soy sauce and sauté.

3. Stir frequently, ensuring you cook all sides of the tempeh cubes.

4. Remove from heat and add the garlic powder, salt, and pepper

NUTRITION FACTS

- Serving Size: 1 ½ cups each Calorie: 268 Sugar: 4 g Sodium: 327 mg Fat: 13 g Saturated Fat: 2 g Carbohydrates: 25 g Fiber: 4 g Protein: 16 g

CHICKEN PARMESAN

YIELD: 4 Servings

Complete Lean and Green Meal: 1 Leaner, 3 Green, 1 Healthy Fat, 3 Condiments

Per Serving: 360 calories, 49g protein, 16g Carbohydrate, 12g Fat

Total Time: 30

INGREDIENTS

- 1¾ lb boneless skinless chicken breasts

- ½ cup almond flour

- 2tbsp + 2tsp large flake nutritional yeast

- ½ tsp each: salt and pepper divided

- 1, 15oz can petite diced tomatoes

- ½ tsp dried oregano

- 2 cloves garlic minced

- 2 scallions, chopped

- 2 medium zucchini (1lb total), cut, sliced, or "sparlized" into noodle-like strands (should yield about 4 cups zucchini noodles)

DIRECTIONS

1. Preheat oven to 400°F

2. Combine almond flour and nutritional yeast in a medium sized bowl—season chicken breast with salt and pepper, the coat both sides with almond mixture.

3. Bake for 12 to 15 minutes or until internal temperature reaches 165°F. Once cooked, remove chicken from the oven and set aside to rest.

4. While chicken bakes, combine tomatoes, oregano, garlic and scallions in a pot and simmer on low for 15 to 20 minutes.

5. Steam zucchini "noodles" in a steamer basket over boiling water on stovetop until tender.

6. Serve zucchini "noodles" with marinara and chicken.

HOMEMADE BEAN DIP

Makes: 1 ½ cups

Time: 27 minutes (5 minutes prep time, 12 minutes cook time, 10 minutes natural release) + overnight bean soak

Homemade bean dip is very easy and delicious with fresh-cut veggies, pita, or pita chips. This recipe produces 1 ½ cups, so make this for you and a movie-night buddy to share. Keep in mind that you'll need to soak the beans overnight before using the pressure cooker.

INGREDIENTS:

- 3 cups of water
- 2 cups soaked split fava beans
- 2 crushed garlic cloves
- 2 tablespoons veggie oil
- 1 tablespoon olive oil
- 1 zested and juiced lemon
- 2 teaspoons tahini
- 2 teaspoons cumin
- 1 teaspoon harissa
- 1 teaspoon paprika
- Salt to taste

DIRECTIONS

1. The night before, soak the fava beans and drain the fava beans before beginning the recipe.
2. Preheat your pressure cooker.
3. Add garlic when hot and cook until they become golden.
4. Add beans, veggie oil, and 3 cups of water.
5. Close and seal the lid.

6. Select "manual" and cook on high pressure for 12 minutes.

7. When time is up, hit "cancel" and wait 10 minutes before quickly releasing any remaining pressure.

8. Drain the cooking liquid from the pressure cooker, leaving about 1 cup.

9. Toss in the tahini, cumin, harissa, and lemon zest.

10. Puree until smooth.

11. Salt and blend again.

12. Serve with a drizzle of olive oil and dash of paprika.

NUTRITION FACTS

➢ Total calories: 415

➢ Protein: 15

➢ Carbs: 31

➢ Fiber: 7

➢   Fat: 26

MANGO CHUTNEY

Serving: 2 cups

Time: 25 minutes (5 minutes prep time, 20 minutes cook time)

Mango chutney is a spicy-sweet condiment used in everything from curries to sandwiches with avocado and alfalfa sprouts. It would also be awesome on a veggie burger! Cooking Tip: Refrigerated chutney will last up to a month, while in the freezer, it can last up to a year.

INGREDIENTS:

- 2 big, diced mangos
- 1 cored and diced apple
- 1 ¼ cups apple cider vinegar
- 1 ¼ cups raw sugar
- ¼ cup raisins
- 1 chopped shallot
- 2 tablespoons finely-diced ginger
- 1 tablespoon veggie oil
- 2 teaspoons salt
- ½ teaspoon red pepper flakes
- ¼ teaspoon cardamom powder
- ⅛ tea spoon cinnamon

DIRECTIONS

1. Preheat your pressure cooker
2. When hot, add the oil and cook shallots and ginger until the shallot is soft
3. Add cinnamon, chili powder, and cardamom and cook for 1 minute
4. Add the rest of the ingredients and mix
5. When the sugar has melted, close and seal the lid
6. Select "manual" and cook for 7 minutes on high pressure
7. When the beeper sounds, hit "cancel" and wait for the pressure to come down on its own

8. Turn the pot back to "sauté" with the lid off until the chutney has a jam-like texture

9. When it starts to thicken, turn the cooker to the "keep warm" setting

10. When you get the texture you want, move the chutney to glass jars and close

11. When the contents are cool, move to the fridge.

NUTRITION FACTS (1 tablespoon):

- Total calories: 78.2

- Protein: 9

- Carbs: 18.3

- Fiber: 1

- Fat: 3

MUSHROOM RISOTTO

Serves: 4-6

Time: 30 minutes (10 minutes prep time, 20 minutes cook time)

Rich roasted mushrooms, vegan butter, and umami miso paste make for one delicious risotto. It's so good and satisfying you could eat this as a main course if you wanted, though a small amount as a side dish with stuffed eggplant would also be good.

INGREDIENTS:

- 4 cups veggie stock

- 1 ½ pound mixed, chopped mushrooms

- 1 ounce dried porcini mushrooms
- 2 cups Arborio rice
- 1 cup chopped yellow onion
- ¾ cups dry white wine
- 4 tablespoons olive oil
- 4 tablespoons vegan butter
- 1 tablespoon miso paste
- 2 teaspoons soy sauce
- 2 teaspoons minced garlic
- ½ cup chopped herbs

DIRECTIONS

- Microwave the dried mushrooms in broth for 5 minutes
- Chop the porcini and set aside for now. Keep the broth separate
- Heat olive oil in your pressure cooker
- Add the fresh mixed mushrooms and cook for about 8 minutes until brown
- Season with salt and pepper
- Add the onion, garlic, porcini, and butter
- Stir until the onions are soft
- Add the rice and stir to coat in oil
- When toasty after 3-4 minutes, add the soy sauce and miso paste

- Pour in the wine and cook for 2 minutes

- Pour the broth through a strainer into the pot and deglaze

- Close and seal the pressure cooker

- Select "manual" and cook on high pressure for 5 minutes

- When the beeper goes off, hit "cancel" and quick-release

- Open the lid and stir. If it's not thick enough, turn on the "sauté" program and stir

- Add herbs and season with salt and pepper before serving.

NUTRITION FACTS (⅙ RECIPE):

Total calories: 431

Protein: 10

Carbs: 58

Fiber: 8

Fat: 17

SMOKY LIMA BEANS

Serves: 12 Time: 1 hour, 10 minutes (25 minutes cook time, 5 minutes natural pressure release, 10 minutes boil time, 20-30 minutes simmer time)

For smoky, campfire-ready lima beans, all you need is the right seasonings. No meat at all. For the liquid smoke, Colgin is a good vegan brand, but most brands should be vegan. Just take a look at the ingredient list to be sure. To make enough beans for 12 people, you'll need an 8-quart cooker.

INGREDIENTS

- 12 cups water
- 2 pounds dry large lima beans
- ⅛ cup Colgin liquid smoke
- 1 teaspoon onion powder
- 1 teaspoon garlic powder
- Salt and pepper to taste

DIRECTIONS

1. Rinse beans before putting them into the pressure cooker with your water
2. Add onion and garlic powder, and seal the lid
3. Hit "Bean" and adjust to 25 minutes
4. When time is up, wait 5 minutes and then quick-release the pressure
5. Add salt and liquid smoke
6. Taste and add more seasonings if necessary
7. Hit "sauté" and bring to a boil for 10 minutes
8. Then, hit "cancel."
9. Turn back to "sauté" and simmer for 20-30 minutes, until thickened.

NUTRITION FACTS (½ CUP PER SERVING):

- Total calories: 213

- Protein: 16

- Carbs: 40

- Fat: 0

- Fiber: 7

POLENTA WITH HERBS (OIL FREE)

Time: 20 minutes (5 minutes prep time, 5 minutes cook time, 10 minutes natural release)

Polenta can be tricky to get just right, but it's easy when you use the pressure cooker. This is a simple recipe with simple, rustic flavors from lots of fresh herbs, onion, and garlic. You can use dried; just remember to reduce the amount by about half, since dried herbs have a more concentrated flavor.

Serve: 4-6

INGREDIENTS

- Total calories: 103

- Protein: 0

- Carbs: 3

- Fat: 0

- Fiber: 2

- 4 cups veggie broth

- 1 cup water

- 1 cup coarse-ground polenta

- 1 large minced onion

- 4 tablespoons fresh, chopped thyme

- 2 tablespoons fresh, chopped Italian parsley
- 1 tablespoon minced garlic
- 1 teaspoon fresh, chopped sage
- Salt and pepper to taste

DIRECTIONS

1. Preheat your cooker and dry sauté the onion for about a minute
2. Add the minced garlic and cook for one more minute
3. Pour in the broth, along with the thyme, parsley, and sage
4. Stir
5. Sprinkle the polenta in the pot, but don't stir it in
6. Close and seal the lid
7. Select "manual" and cook on high pressure for 5 minutes
8. When the timer beeps, hit "cancel" and wait 10 minutes
9. Pick out the bay leaf
10. Using a whisk, stir the polenta to smooth it. If it's thin, simmer on the "sauté" setting until it reaches the consistency you like. Season to taste with salt and pepper before serving.

NUTRITION FACTS:

- Polenta calories: 177kcal
- Polenta protein: 3.5g
- Fat: 0.15g

- Carbohydrates: 39g

- Sugar: 0.2g

- Fiber: 2.4g

SWEET THAI COCONUT RICE (OIL FREE)

Time: About 23 minutes (3 minutes cook time, 10 minutes natural release, 5- 10 minutes rest time)

This 5-ingredient side dish can be easily adapted into a dessert by adding more sugar, but it also makes a tasty afternoon snack when you're craving something a little sweet.

INGREDIENTS

- 1 ½ cups water 1 cup Thai sweet rice ½ can full-fat coconut milk

- 2 tablespoons sugar

- Dash of salt

DIRECTIONS

1. Mix rice and water in your pressure cooker

2. Select "manual" and cook for just 3 minutes on high pressure

3. When time is up, hit "cancel" and wait 10 minutes for a natural release

4. In the meanwhile, heat coconut milk, sugar, and salt in a saucepan

5. When the sugar has melted, remove it from the heat

6. When the cooker has released its pressure, mix the coconut milk mixture into your rice and stir

7. Put the lid back on and let it rest 5-10 minutes, without returning it to pressure

8. Serve and enjoy!

NUTRITION FACTS (¼ RECIPE):

- Total calories: 269 Protein: 4

- Carbs: 47

- Fiber: 0

- Fat: 8

PORCINI MUSHROOM PATE

Serves: 6-8

Time: 2 hours, 21 minutes (10 minutes prep time, 11 minutes cook time, 2 hours chill time)

Pate is traditionally made with very fatty meat, which is a big no-no for vegans for various reasons. "True" pate is even illegal in many countries because of animal cruelty laws. Luckily, there's none of that going on in this recipe. You use both fresh and dried mushrooms for a rich, earthy spread seasoned simply with shallot, salt, pepper, and a bay leaf.

INGREDIENTS

- 1 pound sliced fresh cremini mushrooms

- 30 grams rinsed dry porcini mushrooms

- 1 cup boiling water

- ¼ cup dry white wine

- 1 bay leaf
- 1 sliced shallot
- 2 tablespoons olive oil
- 1 ½ teaspoons salt
- ½ teaspoon white pepper

DIRECTIONS

1. Place dry porcini mushrooms in a bowl and pour over boiling water
2. Cover and set aside for now
3. Heat 1 tablespoon of oil in your pressure cooker
4. When hot, cook the shallot until soft
5. Add cremini mushrooms and cook until they've turned golden
6. Deglaze with the wine, and let it evaporate
7. Pour in the porcini mushrooms along with their water
8. Toss in salt, pepper, and the bay leaf
9. Close and seal the lid
10. Select "manual" and cook on high pressure for 10 minutes
11. When the timer beeps, hit "cancel" and quick-release
12. Pick out the bay leaf before adding the last tablespoon of oil
13. Puree mixture until smooth
14. Refrigerate in a closed container for at least 2 hours before eating.

NUTRITION FACTS (⅛ RECIPE):

- Total calories: 70

- Protein: 4

- Carbs: 6

- Fiber: 2.6

- Fat: 4

JAPANESE-PUMPKIN RICE

Serves: 2-4

Time: 22 minutes (5 minutes prep time, 7 minutes cook time, 10 minutes natural release)

This unique rice dish is so easy to make. There are no sautéing or multiple cooking steps; you just put everything in your pressure cooker, cook, and eat! Japanese pumpkin is known in America as Kabocha squash. It's a cross between the sweetness of a pumpkin and a sweet potato.

INGREDIENTS

- 2 cups cubed Kabocha squash

- 2 cups (360 ml) rice

- 1 ½ cups water

- 4 drops sesame oil

- 1 tablespoon cooking sake

- 1 teaspoon

- Salt

DIRECTIONS

1. Mix rice, water, sake, sesame oil, and salt in your pressure cooker

2. Add the squash

3. Close and seal the lid

4. Select "manual," and cook on high pressure for 7 minutes

5. When time is up hit "cancel" and wait 10 minutes

6. Quick-release any remaining pressure

7. Stir and serve!

NUTRITION FACTS (¼ RECIPE):

- Total calories: 355

- Protein: 9

- Carbs: 82

- Fiber: 6

- Fat: 4

THAI CHICKPEAS (OIL FREE)

Serves: 6-8

Time: 18 minutes + overnight chickpea soak

This chickpea side dish has all the flavors - sweet, salty, spicy, savory. The coconut milk creates a gorgeous, creamy sauce that's sweetened with the potatoes, salted with the tamari, spiced with curry powder, and freshened up with herbs. It's perfect for cooked chickpeas.

INGREDIENTS

- 1 ½ cups soaked chickpeas
- 4 cups coconut milk
- ¾ pound peeled and chopped sweet potatoes
- 1 cup chopped canned plum tomatoes
- 1 tablespoon mild curry powder
- ¼ cup fresh, minced coriander
- ½ cup fresh, minced basil
- 1 tablespoon tamari
- 1 teaspoon minced garlic

DIRECTIONS

1. The night before, soak the chickpeas in water on the counter
2. When ready, drain and rinse
3. Add chickpeas to your pressure cooker, along with garlic, potatoes, tomatoes, curry powder, coriander, and coconut milk
4. Close and seal the lid
5. Select "manual" and cook on high pressure for 18 minutes
6. When time is up, hit "cancel" and carefully quick-release
7. If the chickpeas are not done, put the lid back on and simmer
8. Add basil and tamari

9. With a wooden spoon, break up the sweet potatoes and stir, so you get a sauce

10. Serve as is or with rice.

NUTRITIONAL FACTS

- Total calories: 104

- Protein: 2

- Carbs: 15

- Fiber: 6.5

- Fat: 4

EASY GARLIC-ROASTED POTATOES

Serves: 4

Time: 27 minutes (10 minutes prep time, 7 minutes cook time, 10 minutes natural release).

This recipe is for baby potatoes roasted in your pressure cooker. The roasting effect is created by browning the outside of the raw potatoes in oil before cooking under pressure. This keeps the skin crisp.

INGREDIENTS

- 2 pounds baby potatoes

- 4 tablespoons veggie oil

- 4 garlic cloves

- ½ cup veggie stock

- 1 rosemary sprig

- Salt and pepper to taste

DIRECTIONS

1. Preheat your pressure cooker

2. When hot, add oil

3. When the oil is hot, put in your potatoes, garlic, and rosemary

4. Stir to coat the potatoes in oil, and brown on all sides

5. After 8-10 minutes of browning, stop stirring, and pierce the middle of each potato with a knife

6. Pour in the stock

7. Close and seal the lid

8. Select "manual" and cook on high pressure for 7 minutes

9. When time is up, hit "cancel" and wait 10 minutes before quickly releasing any leftover pressure. 10. Season before serving!

NUTRITION FACTS (¼ RECIPE):

- Total calories: 336
- Protein: 5
- Carbs: 49
- Fiber: 7
- Fat: 14

PEANUT BUTTER & PROTEIN PANCAKES

Servings: 1

Prep Time: 5 minutes

Cooking Time: 5 minutes (Per Serving)

- Calories: 397

- Protein: 33 grams

- Carbohydrates: 51 grams

- Fat: 7 grams

INGREDIENTS

- 1/2 banana, mashed

- 2 teaspoons peanut butter

- 1 serving protein powder (of your choice)

- 1/3 cup whole grain pancake batter

- 1 teaspoon honey.

DIRECTIONS

1. In a large mixing bowl, add the banana, peanut butter, protein powder, and batter and mix well.

2. Coat a large nonstick skillet in cooking spray and place over medium heat. Divide the batter evenly in half and spoon onto the skillet.

3. Cook, turning when tops are covered with bubbles and edges look cooked. Drizzle honey on top.

TEX-MEX TOFU TACOS

Servings: 4 (2 tacos per serving)

Prep Time: 5 – 10 minutes

Cooking Time: 15 minutes (Per Serving)

- Calories: 286

- Protein: 16 grams
- Carbohydrates: 26 grams
- Fat: 9 grams

INGREDIENTS

- 2 (14 ounce) packages soft tofu, drained
- 3 (6 inch) corn tortillas, cut into strips
- 1/8 teaspoon turmeric
- 1 jalapeño, seeded and diced
- 1/2 teaspoon smoked paprika
- 4 scallions, trimmed and chopped
- 1/2 teaspoon salt
- 1/4 cup fresh cilantro, chopped
- 2 plum tomatoes, diced
- 1/4 cup vegan cheese, shredded
- 8 (6 inches) corn tortillas, warmed
- 1/2 cup salsa (optional)

DIRECTIONS

1. Coat a large nonstick skillet in cooking spray and place over medium heat. Add the tortilla strips and sauté until golden and crispy, around 6 minutes.

2. Transfer to a plate and set aside. Recoat the pan in cooking spray. Add the tofu to the pan and crumble it into various sized pieces similar to scrambled eggs.

3. Add the turmeric, jalapeño, paprika, scallions, and salt and stir until well combined.

4. Cook until the remaining water in the tofu has cooked off and it has a tender consistency, about 4 – 6 minutes.

5. Add the cilantro, tomatoes, cheese, and tortilla strips. Stir until well combined. Continue stirring until cheese has melted, around 2 minutes.

6. Divide into 4 equal portions, then divide each portion between 2 corn tortillas. Top each taco with 1 tablespoon salsa.

Serve and Enjoy!

MOCHA OATMEAL

Servings: 1

Cooking Time: 5 minutes (Per Serving)

- Calories: 170 Protein: 6 grams

- Carbohydrates: 30 grams

- Fat: 3 grams

INGREDIENTS

- 1/2 cup old-fashioned oats

- 1/2 cup water

- 1/4 cup brewed coffee

- 1 tablespoon unsweetened cocoa powder

- 1 teaspoon stevia or another natural sweetener

DIRECTIONS

1. Cook oats according to package directions.
2. Mix in coffee, cocoa powder and stevia.

QUINOA POWER MUFFINS

Servings: 12 (1 muffin per serving)

Prep Time: 10 minutes

Cooking Time: 20 – 22 minutes (Per Serving)

- Calories: 319
- Protein: 10 grams
- Carbohydrates: 45 grams
- Fat: 17 grams

INGREDIENTS

- 1 1/2 cups all-purpose flour
- 2 teaspoons baking powder
- 1/2 teaspoon baking soda
- 2 packets stevia or other natural sweetener
- 2 teaspoons cinnamon
- 1/2 teaspoon salt
- 3/4 cup wheat bran
- 1/4 cup oat bran
- 3 tablespoons ground flax seed
- 1 1/3 cups almond milk

- 1/3 cup canola oil

- 1 teaspoon vanilla extract

- 1 cup quinoa, cooked

- 1/2 cup walnuts, chopped

- 1/2 cup vegan chocolate chips

- 1/2 cup hemp seeds

DIRECTIONS

1. Preheat oven to 400°F. Coat a 12-cup muffin pan in cooking spray.

2. In a large mixing bowl, add the flour, baking powder, baking soda, stevia, cinnamon, and salt. Whisk together, then pour in the wheat bran, oat bran, and flax seed and whisk until thoroughly combined.

3. In a separate bowl, add the almond milk, canola oil, and vanilla extract. Whisk together, then pour in the quinoa and whisk to combine.

4. Pour the dry ingredients in and mix them together with a wooden or plastic spoon. Fold in the walnuts, chocolate chips, and hemp seeds.

5. Be careful not to over-mix, there should still be some chunks. 4. Pour the batter into the muffin pan, only filling each cup to 3/4 full.

6. Place in oven and bake for 20 – 22 minutes, or until a toothpick inserted into the middle comes out clean.

PESTO ZUCCHINI NOODLES WIGH GRILLED CHICKEN

YIELD: 4 Servings

Per Serving: 1 Leaner, 1 Healthy Fat, 3 Green, 3 Condiment

Total Time: 20- 25 Minutes

INGREDIENTS

- ⅓ cup reduced-fat Italian salad dressing
- ½ cup chopped fresh basil
- ½ parmesan cheese, divided
- ⅓ oz pine nut
- Cooking Spray
- 2 medium to large zucchini (about 1½ lbs), cut, sliced, and "spiralized" into noodle-like strands (should yield 4 cups zucchini noodles)
- 1½ lbs grilled boneless skinless chicken breast, cubed or cut into strips
- 2 cups cherry tomatoes, halved
- ½ tsp crushed red pepper flakes (optional)

DIRECTIONS

1. To make pesto, combine the salad dressing, basil, 2 tablespoons parmesan cheese, and pine nuts in a food processor. Blend until smooth.

2. In a lightly greased skillet over medium heat, cook zucchini noodles until just tender about 3 to 5 minutes. Stir in pesto and remaining parmesan cheese, then remove from heat.

3. Add tomatoes, top with grilled chicken and garnish with crushed red pepper flakes.

NUTRITION FACTS

- 45% Total Fat 29g. 45% Saturated Fat 9g.

- 47% Cholesterol 140mg. 96% Sodium 2310mg.

- 6% Total Carbohydrates 18g. 20% Sugars 9g. Protein 39g.

INSTANT POT CHICKEN TIKKA MASALA

YIELD: 4 Servings

PER SERVING: 1 Leaner, 1 Healthy Fat, 3 Green, 3 Condiments

Total Time: 30 Minutes

INGREDIENTS

- 1, 14-5oz can diced tomatoes

- ½ cup full fat canned coconut milk

- 2 tsp gram masala

- 1 tsp Cumin

- 1 tsp grated fresh ginger

- ½ tsp onion powder

- ½ tsp garlic powder

- ½ smoked paprika

- ¼ tsp turmeric

- ¼ tsp cayenne

- ½ tsp salt

- 1½ lbs boneless skinless chicken thighs, cubed
- 4 cups frozen riced cauliflower
- ¼ cup chopped fresh cilantro

DIRECTIONS

1. Combine the first 11 ingredients in a medium sized bowl.
2. Place chicken in instant Pot and pour sauce over top.
3. Secure lid and close pressure valve. Set to 20 minutes at high pressure. Allow pressure to release naturally before opening.
4. Meanwhile, microwave riced cauliflower according to package directions.
5. To serve: Divide riced cauliflower and chicken evenly amongst 4 bowls. Garnish with cilantro.

NUTRITION FACTS:

SERVING: 1(of 6), about 5/6 cup with 1/2 prepared brown rice

CALORIES: 355kcal CARBOHYDRATES: 32g PROTEIN: 36g FAT: 10g

SATURATED FAT: 5g CHOLESTEROL: 79mg FIBER: 4g

SUGAR: 5g

PB&J OATMEAL

Servings: 4

Prep Time: Under 3 minutes

Cooking Time: 5 – 10 minutes (Per Serving)

- Calories: 376

- Protein: 32 grams

- Carbohydrates: 38 grams

- Fat: 11 grams.

INGREDIENTS

- 1/3 cup old-fashioned oats

- 2/3 cup water

- 1 scoop protein powder (of your choice)

- 1/2 teaspoon vanilla extract

- 1 tablespoon peanut butter

- 1 tablespoon jelly

DIRECTIONS

1. Add the oats and water to a small saucepan and bring to a boil over medium-high heat.

2. Reduce heat to medium-low and let simmer until 90% of the water is absorbed.

3. Remove from the heat, add the protein powder and vanilla extract.

4. Whisk together until well combined. Pour oatmeal into a bowl and top with peanut butter and jelly.

5. Enjoy and Serve!

BIBIMBAP BOWLS

YIELD: 4 Servings

PER SERVING: 1 Leaner, 1 Healthy Fat, 3 Green, 2 Condiments.

Total Time: 15- 20 Minutes

INGREDIENTS

- 1 tsp olive oil
- 5 cups baby spinach
- 1 tsp toasted sesame oil
- ¼ tsp salt
- 1 lb 95-97% lean ground beef
- 2 Tsbpchilli garlic sauce
- 1 Tbsp reduced sodium soy sauce
- 2 cups diced cauliflower
- 1 cup thinly sliced cucumber
- 4 fried or hard-boiled eggs
- ½ cup chopped green onions
- 1 Tbsp sesame seeds

DIRECTIONS

1. Heat the olive oil in a skillet over medium-high heat.

2. Add the spinach, and cook for a few minutes or until just wilted. Drizzle the sesame oil over the top, and lightly season with salt. Remove spinach from skillet, and st aside.

3. Add the ground beef to the skillet used to cook the spinach. Cook the beef until fully browned. Stir in the

chili garlic sauce and soy sauce, cook for one minute, and then remove skillet from heat.

4. Steam the riced cauliflower in the microwave with one tablespoon water until tender, about 3 to 4 minutes.

5. Build the bowls by first adding a ½ cup of riced cauliflower to each one. Arrange a quarter of each on top: spinach, ground beef, and cucumber. Add an egg to each bowl, and garnish with green onions and sesame seeds.

NUTRITION FACTS

1. Calories 772 Calories from Fat 225.

2. Fat 25g38% Saturated Fat 42g263% Cholesterol 233mg78%

3. Sodium 1708mg74% Potassium 1361mg39% Carbohydrates 35g12% Fiber 6g25%

PAD THAI ZUCCHINI NOODLES

YIELD: 4 Servings

PER SERVING: 1 Leaner, 3 Green, 3 Condiments, 1 Healthy Fat

Total Time: 35 Minutes

INGREDIENTS

For Peanut Sauce:

- ½ powdered peanut butter

- 2 Tbsp lime juice

- 1 Tbsp lime zest

- 2 Tbsp low-sodium soy sauce

- 2 tsp grated fresh ginger

- ½ tsp red pepper flakes

- 2-3 Tbsp water (to the thin sauce)

For Zucchini Noodles:

- 4 medium zucchini

- 2 tsp olive oil

- Cooking Spray

- 2 lb raw shrimp, peeled and deveined

- 1 cup chopped or sliced bell pepper

- ½ cup chopped scallions

- 3 whole eggs

- ½ cup bean sprouts

- ½ cup fresh cilantro

- 2 Tbsp sesame seeds, preferably black

DIRECTIONS

1. Combine peanut sauce ingredients in a small bowl, and set aside.

2. Prepare zucchini noodles using a mandolin, julienne peeler or spiralizer.

3. Heat olive oil in a large skillet over medium-high heat. Add zucchini noodles and cook, occasionally stirring, for 2 to 3 minutes. Remove the noodles from the pan, and drain the excess water.

4. Heat a separate large sauté pan over medium-high heat, and lightly grease with cooking spray. Add the shrimp, and cook until the shrimp is tender and becomes pink, about 3 to 4 minutes.

5. Add the bell pepper and green onion and cook for about 1 to 2 minutes until tender. Add the eggs and stir in with the vegetables until the eggs are cooked.

6. Add the zucchini noodles back into the same pan, and then add the sauce. Cook for about 1 more minute, until the zucchini noodles are heated through. Stir in the bean sprouts, cilantro, and sesame seeds, and serve immediately.

NUTRITION FACTS

Serving size: ½ Recipe Calories: 465 Fat: 25 g Saturated fat: 3 g Unsaturated fat: 11 g Trans fat: 0 g Carbohydrates: 45 g Fiber: 6 g Protein: 41 g

BLACK BEAN + QUINOA BURRITOS (VEGAN FREEZER BURRITOS)

Prep Time: 15 min Cook Time: 15 min Total Time: 30 minutes

Yield: Makes 6 - 8 burritos

INGREDIENTS

- ½ cup dried quinoa

- ¾ cup + 1 or 2 tablespoons water

- 1 tablespoon olive oil or ¼ cup water (for water sauté)

- ½ large red onion, diced

- 1 orange bell pepper, seeds removed and diced
- 1 can (14oz) diced tomatoes, drained (or 2 roma tomatoes, seeds removed and diced)
- 1 medium zucchini, diced
- 2 cans (14 oz) black beans, drained and rinsed
- 1 can (14 oz) corn, drained
- ¼ – ½ cup cilantro, roughly chopped
- 2 teaspoons cumin
- 1 teaspoon chili powder
- ¾ – 1 teaspoon chipotle powder or 2 – 4 chipotles in adobe sauce
- 1 teaspoon garlic powder
- ½ teaspoon onion powder
- Mineral salt, to taste
- 6 – 8 medium/large tortillas

INSTRUCTIONS

1. Quinoa: In a small/medium pot, combine the quinoa and water, bring to a boil, cover, reduce heat to low and simmer for 13 minutes. Remove lid, let set 10 minutes, fluff with a fork. Set aside.

2. Filling: In a large pan or pot, heat oil/water over medium heat, add onion and saute for 4 minutes, add bell pepper and continue to cook for 2 minutes. Add the tomatoes, zucchini and corn, cook another 3 minutes or so (cook veggies until they are as soft as you like; I prefer mine to be a little al dente). Add the black beans, quinoa, cilantro, cumin, chipotle, garlic

& onion powder, and salt; continue to cook until heated through.

3. Roll: Place tortillas on a flat surface, place a mound of the filling in the center, leaving room all the way around, fold in half, fold up each end, and roll the burrito away from you to completely close it.

4. Freeze: I try to avoid foil, so here I used paper sandwich bags. Feel free to use foil, freezer paper, saran wrap, plastic freezer Ziploc bags or whatever you're used to freezing with. If using paper sandwich bags, they should be eaten within a few weeks to avoid freezer burn. Most likely they won't be around that long!

5. Reheat: If at room temperature, warm in the oven/toaster oven at 375 degrees F for 10 minutes or so, or microwave for 30 seconds. If frozen heat in the oven at 375 degrees for 30 minutes, or microwave for 1:30 – 2 minutes.

6. Serve with sliced avocado and your favorite salsa

NUTRITION FACTS

Calories: 442kcal | Carbohydrates: 63g | Protein: 20g | Fat: 14g | Saturated Fat: 4g | Cholesterol: 15mg | Sodium: 861mg | Potassium: 711mg | Fiber: 14g | Sugar: 7g | Vitamin A: 1690IU | Vitamin C: 51mg | Calcium: 233mg | Iron: 5mg

VEGAN COCONUT MACAROONS

Toasty coconut on the outside and tender on the inside, these vegan coconut macaroons use minimal ingredients and are super easy to make!

Prep Time: 15 min Cook Time: 25 min Total Time: 40 minutes

Yield: Makes 24

INGREDIENTS

- 3 cups unsweetened coconut flakes, finely shredded (see notes)

- 1 cup canned coconut milk or cream, full or low-fat

- ⅓ cups pure maple syrup

- ⅓ cups slivered almonds (chopped is ok too), optional

- ⅓ cups oat flour, all-purpose, or gluten-free flour blend*

- 2 teaspoons vanilla extract

- Pinch of mineral salt

- 7 oz. vegan dark chocolate bar or chocolate chips

INSTRUCTIONS

- Preheat oven to 350 degrees F. Line a baking sheet with parchment paper or a Silpat.

- Mix: In a medium size mixing bowl, combine the coconut, coconut milk, syrup, almonds, flour, vanilla and salt, mix well.

- Scoop: Using a 2 or 3 tablespoons measuring spoon, scoop out rounded tablespoons, making sure to pack it well. This last part is very important, or your macaroons may tend to fall apart. Place packed mounds on cookie sheet, about 1 inch apart.

- Bake: Place cookie sheet in the oven and bake for 20 – 30 minutes (ovens vary and it depends on how big the mounds are), until golden, rotating sheet halfway through baking. Let cool completely.

- Chocolate: Warm the chocolate on the stove over low heat, frequently stirring until melted. Alternately, you can melt the chocolate in the microwave, stopping to give a good stir every 30 seconds. Dip the bottoms of the macaroons into the melted chocolate. Place the cookies back on the lined baking sheet—drizzle remaining chocolate on top using a spoon or pastry piping bag. Refrigerate for 7 – 10 minutes, or until set.

NUTRITION FACTS

Total Fat 7g 9% Saturated Fat 6.5g 33% Total Carbs 16g 6%

Total Sugars 11g Protein 1g 2%

SIDES AND DINNER

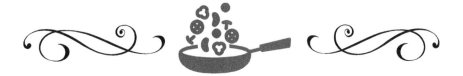

MANGO COCONUT POPSICLES (+ GRANOLA)

Cool off with these mango + coconut popsicles with granola. They can be made in popsicle molds, or small dixie cups for a healthy treat any time of day.

Prep Time: 10 min Cook Time: 6 hours Total Time: 6 hours 10 minutes

Yield: Makes 6 – 10 popsicles

INGREDIENTS

- 2 mangos, cubed or 16 oz. bag frozen mango, thawed
- 1 lime, juice of
- 1 cup unsweetened canned coconut milk (I recommend Target's Good & Gather)
- 1 – 2 tablespoons pure maple syrup
- ½ cup vegan granola of choice

INSTRUCTIONS

1. Puree: In a blender, mango (about 3 cups), and lime juice, puree until smooth.

2. Combine: Mix the coconut milk and pure maple syrup.

3. Assemble: Pour the mango puree into the mold, about ⅓ full. Add a little granola, gently press down, sinking them a little into the mixture. Pour in a layer of coconut milk. Repeat with another layer of mango puree. Top each mold with a little granola. Tap the molds gently on the counter to remove any excess air bubbles, and place the stick or cut straw right in the center.

4. Freeze: Place in the freezer, towards the back if possible, for at least 6 hours.

5. Remove from molds: Let sit at room temp for a few moments. It should slide out easily or with a little pull. Alternately, place the popsicle maker in room temp water, letting it reach just under the brim of the pop maker. Do this just for a few seconds. Remove popsicles with a gentle pull.

6. Makes about 10 regular-sized popsicles 6 – 4.5 oz. Popsicles.

NUTRITION FACTS

Calories: 200.3kcal Carbohydrates: 36g Protein: 2.3g Fat: 6.7g

Saturated Fat: 5.2g Fiber: 3.8g Sugar: 31.2g Net Carbs: 32.2g

ROASTED POBLANO TACOS

Roasted Poblano Tacos are loaded with protein rich beans, poblano chiles, avocado and cilantro.

Prep Time: 10 min Cook Time: 10 min Total Time: 20 minutes

Yield: Serves 3

INGREDIENTS

- 2 medium poblano chiles (Anaheim or hatch chilies ok too)
- 1 can (15 oz) pinto, black beans or refried beans
- 2 scallions, sliced
- Purple or green cabbage, shredded
- Avocado, sliced
- Cilantro
- 6 corn tortillas (or 9 organic corn tortilla sliders)
- Lime wedges, to serve
- Hatch chile cashew dressing or cilantro lime cashew cream, to serve

INSTRUCTIONS

1. Roast poblanos: Turn broiler to medium – high, place poblanos on baking sheet and place under the broiler for about 7 – 10 minutes, turning every few minutes to char and brown evenly on all sides. Poblanos will crackle and pop while cooking, they will be ready when charred and softened to the touch of a fork pushing on its side. Place poblanos in a bowl, cover with a plate or saran wrap and let steam for a few minutes (this will help loosen the skin for peeling). Remove the skin, lay the peeled poblano on a flat surface, remove the top and make a slit down the

center, open and remove the seeds. Slice lengthwise into ½ inch strips.

2. Heat beans: Place beans in a small pot and cook over medium until warm, stirring occasionally. If using pinto or black beans, add a dash or two garlic powder for a little extra flavor. You may decide not to heat your canned whole beans in which case, drain and rinse before using.

3. Prep veggies: Prepare scallions, purple cabbage and avocado. Heat your tortillas over the gas/electric burner until slightly charred.

4. Build: Layer your tacos with beans, poblanos, cabbage, scallions, avocado, cilantro and a sprinkle of pink salt & drizzle of cashew cream of choice or sriracha (or both!).

NUTRITION FACTS

Calories: 407; Total Fat: 15g; Saturated Fat: 2g; Monounsaturated Fat: 3g; Cholesterol: 0mg; Sodium: 312mg; Carbohydrate: 40g; Dietary Fiber: 7g; Sugar: 6g; Protein: 8g

SOUTHERN BLACKBERRY COBBLER (VEGAN + EASY)

With only 7 ingredients this flavorful vegan blackberry cobbler is a great way to use up the season's abundance of blackberries.

Prep Time: 5 min Cook Time: 35 min Total Time: 40 minutes

Yield: Serves 6

INGREDIENTS

- 1 cup spelled flour
- ½ cup coconut sugar
- 1 tablespoon baking powder
- ½ teaspoon cinnamon
- 1 cup unsweetened vanilla plant milk, warmed if using coconut oil
- ⅓ cups coconut oil or vegan butter/margarine, warmed to a liquid state
- 3 cups fresh or frozen blackberries

INSTRUCTIONS

1. Preheat oven to 350 degrees F.

2. Batter: In a medium bowl, combine flour, sugar, baking powder and cinnamon. Be sure to warm your milk if using coconut oil before using or it will harden the coconut oil when combined. Add milk and mix well. Add oil/butter, mix well again.

3. Assemble: Pour batter into an 8 inch baking dish. Drop blackberries into the batter, distributing evenly all over. You may even push down some of the blackberries into the batter, then add more over the top. Sprinkle a little pure cane sugar over top if you like. I would refrain from using coconut sugar as it may burn. If you want to add coconut sugar, sprinkle some at least halfway through baking time.

4. Bake: Place in oven on the middle rack and bake for 35 – 40 minutes. Let cool a few minutes and serve.

5. Pairs great with a scoop of non-dairy vanilla ice cream for dessert and a scoop of vanilla non-dairy

yogurt for breakfast (yes, this would be a fine way to start your day!)

NUTRITION FACTS

Total Fat 13.5g   17% Saturated Fat 10.1g   Cholesterol
0mg   0%

Sodium 215.6mg   9% Total Carbohydrate 28.3g   10%
Dietary Fiber 7g   25%

Sugars 5.5g   Protein 5.5g 11%

CHUNKY APPLE-CINNAMON OATMEAL BREAKFAST COOKIES

Healthy Chunky Apple-Cinnamon Oatmeal Breakfast Cookies with only 4 ingredients are full of flavor and are best served warm fresh from the oven!

Prep Time: 10 min Cook Time: 20 min Total Time: 30 minutes

Yield: Makes 18

INGREDIENTS

- 2 ½ cups old-fashioned oats (quick-oats or combo is ok too)

- 1 ½ cups unsweetened applesauce

- 2 teaspoons cinnamon

- ½ apple, cored and diced

- ¼ cup organic sugar, + more for sprinkling

INSTRUCTIONS

1. Prep: Preheat oven to 350 degrees F. Line a baking sheet with parchment, a Silpat, or lightly grease with oil.

2. Mix: In a medium size mixing bowl, combine the oats, applesauce, cinnamon, mix well to combine. Prepare the apple, letting the mixture set for a few minutes. Add the apple and mix again.

3. Scoop: Using a tablespoon measurer, scoop out well-rounded mounds of the mixture, making sure to gently pack it with your fingers, place it on a cookie sheet. If these aren't packed well enough they may have a tendency to fall apart. Sprinkle the top of each cookie with sugar, this last step is optional.

4. Bake: Place cookie sheet in the oven, on the middle rack, and bake for 17 – 20 minutes.

NUTRITION FACTS:

Fat 5g8% Saturated Fat 3g19% Cholesterol 22mg7% Sodium 71mg3% Potassium 50mg1% Carbohydrates 19g6% Sugar 9g10% Protein 1g2%

STRAWBERRY + RHUBARB CRISP

A perfect combination of sweet & tart! Easy homemade Strawberry & Rhubarb Crisp is a family favorite! Great have a dessert, but healthy enough for side dishes and dinner.

Prep Time: 10 min Cook Time: 40 min Total Time: 50 minutes

Yield: Serves 4 - 6

INGREDIENTS

- Filling
- 4 – 5 stalks of rhubarb, chopped
- 2 lbs. strawberries, quartered
- 2 tablespoons coconut or cane sugar
- Topping
- 1 ½ cups old fashioned oats (I used GF)
- ½ cup almond meal
- ½ teaspoon cinnamon
- ¼ teaspoon cardamom
- 1 teaspoon vanilla extract
- ¼ cup coconut or cane sugar (maple syrup works too)
- ⅓ cups coconut oil, room temperature or any neutral oil
- ⅓ – ½ cup slivered almonds (chopped walnuts or pecans work too)
- Pinch of mineral salt

INSTRUCTIONS

1. Preheat oven to 350 degrees F.
2. Using a 9×9 baking dish, add rhubarb and strawberries directly to the dish, add sugar, and mix gently.
3. In a medium size bowl, mix together the ingredients for the topping. Spread evenly over the top of the strawberries & rhubarb mixture.

4. Bake on the middle rack for 40 – 50 minutes. It Will be done when the mixture is bubbly and top is golden. Let cool for 10 minutes.

5. Serve warm with a dollop of non-dairy vanilla yogurt or a scoop of your favorite non-dairy vanilla ice cream.

NUTRITION FACTS

Per 1/12 of recipe 210 calories 3 grams of protein 23 grams of carbohydrates 4 grams of fiber 6 milligrams of sodium 320 milligrams of potassium 15 milligrams of cholesterol

VEGAN BLACK BEAN ENCHILADAS

Description: A mixture of black beans, vegetables, and spices make these enchiladas a hearty, delicious dinner. They have no meat or dairy, but they're plenty flavorful and will be sure to fill you up.

Servings: 6

INGREDIENTS

- 2 cans red enchilada sauce (10 oz. per can)
- 1/2 red onion (medium)
- 1 red bell pepper (medium)
- 1 jalapeno pepper (small, optional)
- 2 garlic cloves
- 1 tablespoon extra-virgin olive oil
- 1 can black beans (13.5 oz. per can, drained and rinsed)

- 1 can Hatch mild diced green chiles (4 oz. per can)

- 1/2 teaspoon salt

- 1/4 teaspoon black pepper

- 1 teaspoon ground cumin

- 1 teaspoon ground coriander

- 1/2 teaspoon dried oregano

- 12 soft corn tortillas (6-inch diameter)

- Fresh cilantro (optional, for garnish)

NUTRITION FACTS:

- Total Fat 36.2g 46% Saturated Fat 6.8g   Trans   Fat 0g Polyunsaturated Fat 3.2g

- Monounsaturated Fat 15.3g 0% Cholesterol 30mg 10% Sodium 1450.2mg 63%

- Total Carbohydrate 73.3g 27% Dietary Fiber 20.3g 73% Sugars 9.6g Protein 26.3g 53%

LEMON GARLIC OREGANO CHICKEN WITH ASPARAGUS

YIELD: 4 Servings

PER SERVING: 1 Lean, 3 Green, 2 Condiments

Total Time: 45 Minutes

INGREDIENTS

- 1¾ lbs bone-in, skinless chicken thighs

- 1 small lemon, juiced (about 2 tbsp lemon juice)

- 2 cloves garlic, minced

- 2 tbsp fresh oregano, minced

- ¼ tsp each (or less) salt and black pepper

- 2lbs asparagus, trimmed

DIRECTIONS

1. Pre-heat oven to 350°F

2. Add the chicken to a medium-sized bowl. Add the lemon juice, garlic, oregano, salt and pepper, and toss to combine.

3. Roast chicken in the oven until it reaches an internal temperature of 165°F, about 40 minutes. Once the chicken thighs are cooked, remove and set aside to rest.

4. Meanwhile, steam asparagus on a stovetop or in the microwave to the desired doneness.

5. Serve asparagus with roasted chicken thighs.

NUTRITION FACTS:

- per serving Serves 4

- Calories 302, Total C 7.9g, Fiber 1.8g, Net C 6.1g, Sugar 2.7g, Fat 16.9g, Protein 31.1g

VEGGIE CHIPS AND BUFFALO CHICKEN DIPS

YIELD: 4 Servings

PER SERVING: 1 Leaner, 3 Green, 1 Healthy Fat, 3 Condiments

Total Time: 55 Minutes

INGREDIENTS

FOR VEGGIE CHIPS

- 1 Tbsp olive oil
- 2 tsp lemon juice
- ½ tsp salt
- ½ tsp pepper
- ½ tsp rosemary
- 3 cups thinly sliced yellow squash
- 3 cups thinly sliced zucchini

FOR BUFFALO CHICKEN DIP:

- 4 light spreadable cheese wedges, softened
- 1½ cup plain, low-fat Greek yogurt
- ¼ cup light ranch dressing
- ¼ cup hot pepper sauce
- 1, 12.5oz can chicken breast, drained
- 1 cup moderate-fat, shredded Colby and Monterey Jack cheese
- Cooking spray

DIRECTIONS

- Preheat oven to 400°F
- Whisk the olive oil, lemon juice, salt, pepper, and rosemary together in a large mixing bowl.
- Add yellow squash and zucchini, and gently mix to coat.

- On a large, lightly greased baking sheet, arrange yellow squash and zucchini slices in a single layer.

- Bake for 20 to 30 minutes, until crisp.

- Meanwhile, mix all dip ingredients until smooth, and transfer the dip mixture to a small, lightly greased baking dish.

- Once chips are removed from the oven, add dip mixture and bake for 15 to 20 minutes, until lightly browned, hot and bubbling.

NUTRITION FACTS

Calories: 340 Fat: 14g Carbohydrates: 15g Protein: 35g

CHEESE STUFFED PORTABELLA MUSHROOMS

YIELD: 2 Servings

PER SERVING: 1 Lean, 3 Green, 2 Condiments

Total Time: 25 Minutes

INGREDIENTS

- 4 large portabella mushroom caps, stemmed

- 1 Tbsp lemon juice

- 1 Tbsp soy sauce

- 1 tsp olive oil, divided

- 2 cups reduced-fat, shredded mozzarella cheese

- ½ cup chopped fresh tomato

- ½ tsp Italian seasoning

- 1 clove garlic, minced
- 1 Tbsp chopped fresh cilantro

DIRECTIONS

1. Preheat oven to 400°F

2. Using a spoon, scoop out the interior of mushroom caps to create "bowls."

3. In a small bowl, combine lemon juice, soy sauce and half of the olive oil. Brush both sides of the mushroom caps with mixture. Place onto a foil lined baking sheet, and bake until soft, about 10 to 12 minutes.

4. Meanwhile, in a medium-sized bowl, combine mozzarella, tomatoes, Italian seasoning, garlic and remaining olive oil.

5. Divide cheese mixture evenly amongst the mushrooms caps, and bake until cheese is melted, an additional 5 to 7 minutes.

6. Serve topped with cilantro.

NUTRITION FACTS

Calories: 196 cal, Fat: 10g, Protein: 13g, Carbohydrate: 14g, Sugar: 6g, Fiber: 3g, Sodium: 567mg

ASIAN GINGER BROCCOLI

Servings: 4

Prep Time: Under 5 mins

Cooking Time: 6 mins (Per Serving)

INGREDIENTS

- 1 tablespoon canola oil
- 2 tablespoons minced garlic
- 4 teaspoons fresh ginger, minced
- 5 cups broccoli crowns, halved
- 3 tablespoons water
- 1 tablespoon rice vinegar

DIRECTIONS

1. Heat the oil in a large skillet over medium-high heat. Add the garlic and ginger and sauté until fragrant, about 45 seconds. Add the broccoli and sauté until broccoli is bright green, about 2 minutes.

2. Pour in the water, stir and cover. Reduce heat to medium and cook until broccoli is tender, about 3 minutes. Toss with vinegar.

NUTRITION FACTS

- Calories: 73
- Protein: 4 grams
- Carbohydrates: 8 grams
- Fat: 4 grams

SAUTÉED CAULIFLOWER

Servings: 4

Prep Time: Under 5 mins Cooking Time: 10 mins

(Per Serving) Calories: 38 Protein: 3 grams Carbohydrates: 8 grams Fat: 0 grams

INGREDIENTS

- 4 cups cauliflower florets, chopped
- 2 tablespoons water
- 2 teaspoons red wine vinegar
- 1 cup grape tomatoes, halved
- 2 tablespoons fresh parsley, chopped
- 1 tablespoon minced garlic
- 1/4 teaspoon salt
- 1/4 teaspoon ground black pepper

DIRECTIONS

1. Coat a large nonstick skillet in cooking spray and place over medium heat. Add the cauliflower, cover and cook for 4 minutes, stirring occasionally.

2. Pour in the water and vinegar, stir to combine and cover. Let cook until cauliflower is golden and tender and the liquid has evaporated, about 4 more minutes.

3. Add the tomatoes, parsley, garlic, salt, and pepper. Cook until tomatoes have softened and flavors have combined, about 2 more minutes.

GARLIC ROSEMARY MUSHROOMS

Servings: 4

Prep Time: Under 5 mins

Cooking Time: 10 mins

INGREDIENTS

- 1 pound mixed mushrooms, cut into 1/4-inch slices
- 2 cloves garlic, finely chopped
- 1/2 tablespoon fresh rosemary, chopped
- 1/4 teaspoon salt
- 1/8 teaspoon ground black pepper
- 1/4 cup dry white wine

DIRECTIONS

1. Coat a large skillet in cooking spray and place over medium heat. Add the mushrooms, garlic, rosemary, salt, and pepper.

2. Cook until mushrooms are soft, about 8 minutes, stirring occasionally. Pour in the wine and stir, cook until mostly evaporated, 1 – 2 minutes.

NUTRITION FACTS (Per Serving):

- Calories: 52
- Protein: 6 grams
- Carbohydrates: 7 grams
- Fat: 1 gram

MEDITERRANEAN BROCCOLI

Servings: 4

Prep Time: 5 mins

Cooking Time: 10 – 12 mins

INGREDIENTS

- 4 cups broccoli florets
- 1 cup cherry tomatoes
- 1 tablespoon extra-virgin olive oil
- 2 cloves garlic, minced
- 1/4 teaspoon salt
- 1/2 teaspoon lemon zest
- 1 tablespoon lemon juice
- 1/4 cup black olives, pitted and sliced
- 1 teaspoon dried oregano
- 2 teaspoons capers, rinsed

DIRECTIONS

1. Preheat oven to 450°F. Coat a baking sheet in cooking spray.

2. In a large mixing bowl, add the broccoli, tomatoes, olive oil, garlic, and salt and toss to coat. Spread out on the baking sheet and bake until broccoli begins to brown, 10 – 12 minutes.

3. Meanwhile, take the large mixing bowl and add the lemon zest, lemon juice, olives, oregano, and capers. Add the cooked vegetables and stir to combine.

NUTRITION FACTS

- (Per Serving):
- Calories: 85
- Protein: 2 grams

- Carbohydrates: 8 grams
- Fat: 4 grams

ASPARAGUS STIR-FRY

Servings: 4

Prep Time: Under 5 mins

Cooking Time: 8 – 10 mins

INGREDIENTS

- 1/4 medium onion, chopped
- 1 pound fresh asparagus, trimmed
- 1 clove garlic, thinly sliced
- 2 teaspoons teriyaki sauce

DIRECTIONS

1. Coat a large skillet in cooking spray and place over medium heat. Add the onions and sauté until tender, 1 – 2 minutes.

2. Add the asparagus and garlic and sauté for 3 – 5 minutes, until asparagus is slightly tender. Pour in the teriyaki sauce and stir for an additional minute to let the flavors combine.

NUTRITION FACTS

(Per Serving): Calories: 30 Protein: 3 grams

Carbohydrates: 6 grams Fat: 0 grams

EGGPLANT "BACON"

Servings: 4 Prep Time: 1 hour, including marination

Cooking Time: 45 mins

INGREDIENTS

- 1 large eggplant, sliced lengthwise into 1/4-inch thick (or less) slices
- 2 tablespoons tamari
- 2 tablespoons maple syrup
- 2 tablespoons apple cider vinegar
- 2 tablespoons extra-virgin olive oil
- 1 teaspoon chili powder
- 1/4 teaspoon smoked paprika
- 1/8 teaspoon ground black pepper

DIRECTIONS

1. Place all of the ingredients in a large ziplock bag, seal and shake to coat. Place in refrigerator and marinate for at least an hour.

2. Preheat oven to 350°F.

3. Lay slices out on a baking sheet and bake, occasionally basting with the marinade, for about 45 minutes or until the desired level of crispiness.

NUTRITION FACTS:

Calories 26.4 Potassium 104.7 mg   Total Carbohydrate 3.3 g
Dietary Fiber 1.2 g   Sugars 0.2 g

CARROT FRIES

Servings: 1 Prep Time: Under 5 mins

Cooking Time: 40 – 45 mins

INGREDIENTS

- 2 large carrots, cut into fry shape wedges
- 1 teaspoon coconut oil
- 1/4 teaspoon salt
- 1/8 teaspoon ground black pepper

DIRECTIONS

1. Preheat oven to 450°F. Coat a baking sheet in cooking spray.
2. In a large mixing bowl add all of the ingredients. Toss until well combined. Spread the carrots out on the baking sheet and bake 40 – 45 minutes, or until lightly browned.

NUTRITION FACTS

(Per Serving): Calories: 101 Protein: 1 gram

Carbohydrates: 7 grams Fat: 5 grams

GREEK POTATOES

Servings: 6

Prep Time: Under 5 mins

Cooking Time: 1 hr 30 mins

INGREDIENTS

- 4 large potatoes, peeled and cut into large wedges
- 2 garlic cloves, minced
- 2 tablespoons extra-virgin olive oil
- 1 cup water
- 1 tablespoon dried oregano
- 1 lemon, juiced
- 1/2 teaspoon salt
- 1/4 teaspoon ground black pepper

DIRECTIONS

1. Preheat oven to 420°F. Coat a baking dish in cooking spray.
2. Place all of the ingredients in the baking dish and toss until well combined.
3. Place in oven and bake for 40 minutes, or until a nice golden-brown crust has formed on the potatoes. Remove from oven and stir to bring the white underside up, sprinkle with a little more salt, pepper, and oregano.
4. If the dish is getting dry add another 1/2 cup of water and place back in the oven for another 40 minutes, or until the new top is browned.

NUTRITION FACTS

- (Per Serving):
- Calories: 212

- Protein: 3 grams
- Carbohydrates: 40 grams
- Fat: 5 grams

CREAMY CAULIFLOWER MASH

Servings: 8

Prep Time: 5 mins

 Cooking Time: 20 – 25 mins

INGREDIENTS

- 3 cups cauliflower florets, steamed and chopped
- 1/2 cup cashews, soaked and drained
- 1/4 cup water
- 1 lemon, juiced
- 1/4 teaspoon salt
- 1 1/2 cups millet, cooked

DIRECTIONS

1. In a food processor or blender, add the cashews, water, lemon juice, and salt and process until smooth. Add the cauliflower and continue to process until well combined.

2. Slowly add in the millet and process until desired consistency (I like mine with a little texture).

NUTRITION FACTS

- (Per Serving):

- Calories: 231
- Protein: 7 grams
- Carbohydrates: 34 grams
- Fat: 8 grams

SPICED RED CABBAGE

- Servings: 6
- Prep Time: Under 5 mins
- Cooking Time: 1 hr

INGREDIENTS

- 1/2 medium head red cabbage, diced
- 1 tablespoon canola oil
- 1/2 cup onion, chopped
- 1 medium apple, quartered
- 3 tablespoons tarragon vinegar
- 1 teaspoon stevia or another natural sweetener
- 1 bay leaf
- 1 teaspoon salt
- 1/4 teaspoon ground black pepper
- 1/8 teaspoon ground cloves

DIRECTIONS

1. Add 1 inch of water to a large saucepan and place over medium-high heat. Add the cabbage and bring to a

boil. Reduce heat, cover and simmer for 4 – 5 minutes, until crisp. Drain.

2. Return to pan, add the remaining ingredients and mix well. Cover and simmer for 1 hour or until cabbage is tender. Remove bay leaf before serving.

NUTRITION FACTS

- (Per Serving):
- Calories: 63
- Protein: 2 grams
- Carbohydrates: 11 grams
- Fat: 3 grams

CRANBERRY APRICOT SQUASH

Servings: 4

Prep Time: Under 5 mins

Cooking Time: Under 10 mins

INGREDIENTS

- 1 pound delicata squash, seeded and chopped into bite-sized pieces
- 1 tablespoon extra-virgin olive oil
- 1 tablespoon apple cider
- 1/4 teaspoon salt
- 1/4 teaspoon ground black pepper
- 1/4 cup dried apricots, chopped
- 1/4 cup dried cranberries

- 2 tablespoons chives, finely chopped

- 2 tablespoons sliced almonds, toasted

DIRECTIONS

1. Place a large saucepan with about 1 inch of water over medium-high heat and bring to a boil. Place the squash in a steamer basket and steam until tender, about 5 – 7 minutes.

2. In a large mixing bowl, add the olive oil, apple cider, salt, and pepper and whisk until well combined. Add the squash, apricots, cranberries, and chives and toss to coat. Sprinkle with almonds.

NUTRITION FACTS

- (Per Serving):

- Calories: 175

- Protein: 2 grams

- Carbohydrates: 32 grams

- Fat: 6 grams

SALADS
AND SOUPS

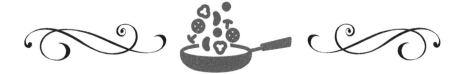

Before we get to some of the smashing salad recipes, few exciting tips will help build an all-rounder salad brimming with all kinds of essential nutrients, and minerals.

a. Go Green

Build a strong foundation before you get to the finer details. So pick lettuce, beans, broccoli and other greens as they'll fare as the most important and healthiest part of your salad. Why go green? Because green foods are a great source of phytonutrients. They help you regulate blood sugar during the day and are packed with fiber and water.

b. Time for Fiber

Lentils and legumes, flax seeds, chia seeds and hemp seeds are rich in fiber and work well in salads. High fiber foods take longer to digest so they keep you full for longer. Fiber also helps with weight loss and maintains the smooth function of the gastric system.

c. Eat More Protein

You can get protein in your diet without having to chow down chicken or fish. Quinoa, buckwheat, soy/tofu, cottage cheese; are all some great options that go well in a salad and in fact compliment all the other seasonal produce you plan to use. Protein helps reduce the risk of cardiovascular diseases and lowers blood pressure.

d. A Handful of Nuts

Nuts lend a great texture to salads. Try almonds, walnuts, pistachio, pine nuts and pecans: all of them work well. Nuts are also a powerhouse of energy, full of natural fiber, proteins, minerals and even unsaturated fats.

e. What's in Season?

Pick the best of what is in the season that will be fresh and flavorful. It'll also be lighter on your budget. This means picking up bright bell peppers, pumpkins, zucchini, mangoes, melons in the summers and cauliflower, peas and the like in the winter.

Salads are a great option for those looking to switch to healthy eating. According to Wayne Campbell, Professor of Nutrition Science at Purdue University in the United States,

"Eating a salad with a variety of colorful vegetables provides several unique types of carotenoids, including beta-carotene, lutein, zeaxanthin and lycopene."

QUINOA & SMOKED TOFU SALAD

Servings: 6

Prep Time: 10 mins

Cooking Time: 20 mins

Cooking Time: 10 – 15 mins

INGREDIENTS

- 1 cup quinoa, rinsed

- 2 cups water

- 3/4 teaspoon salt, divided
- 1/4 cup lemon juice
- 2 tablespoons extra-virgin olive oil
- 2 cloves garlic, minced
- 1/4 teaspoon ground black pepper
- 1 (6 ounces) package baked smoked tofu, diced
- 1 yellow bell pepper, diced
- 1 cup grape tomatoes, halved
- 1 cup cucumber, diced
- 1/2 cup fresh parsley, chopped
- 1/2 cup fresh mint, chopped

DIRECTIONS

1. Add the water and 1/2 teaspoon of salt to a medium saucepan and place over medium-high heat. Bring to a boil, add the quinoa and return to a boil. Reduce to low, cover and cook until water has been fully absorbed, about 15 – 20 minutes.

2. Meanwhile, in a large mixing bowl, add the lemon juice, olive oil, garlic, pepper, and the remaining 1/4 teaspoon of salt. Whisk together until well combined.

3. Spread the quinoa out on a baking sheet to cool for at least 10 minutes. Add the cooled quinoa, tofu, bell pepper, tomatoes, cucumber, parsley, and mint to the dressing. Toss until well coated.

NUTRITION FACTS

(Per Serving):

Calories: 206

Protein: 10 grams

Carbohydrates: 23 grams

Fat: 8 grams

PEAR & QUINOA SALAD

Servings: 6

Prep Time: Under 5 mins

Cooking Time: 15 – 20 mins

INGREDIENTS

- 14 ounces low-sodium vegetable broth
- 1 cup quinoa, rinsed
- 2 tablespoons canola oil
- 1 tablespoon pear or raspberry vinegar
- 1/4 cup fresh chives, diced
- 1/4 teaspoon salt
- 1/4 teaspoon ground black pepper
- 2 medium pears, diced
- 1/8 cup walnuts, chopped

DIRECTIONS

1. Add the vegetable broth to a large saucepan and place over medium-high heat. Once boiling, add the quinoa and reduce heat to medium low to simmer. Stir well and cover with a tight fitting lid. Cook for about 15 minutes, until all the liquid is absorbed.

2. Meanwhile, in a large mixing bowl add the oil, vinegar, chives, salt, and pepper and whisk to combine. Add the pears and toss to coat.

3. Pour the cooked quinoa into the mixing bowl and mix until well combined. Sprinkle nuts over the top. Can be served chilled or warm.

NUTRITION FACTS

- (Per Serving):

- Calories: 231

- Protein: 7 grams

- Carbohydrates: 34 grams

- Fat: 8 grams

BUTTERNUT SQUASH & BLACK BEAN CHILI

Full of fall squash, veggies and hints of chipotle powder and cinnamon, this vegan Butternut Squash & Black Bean Chili make a really excellent warm autumn chili!

Prep Time: 10 min

Cooking Time: 45 minutes

Total Time: 55 minutes

Yield: Serves 4 – 6

INGREDIENTS

- 1 tablespoon olive oil or ¼ cup water, for water, sauté

- 1 medium onion (any color), diced

- cloves garlic, minced (or 1 teaspoon garlic powder)
- 1 heaping Tablespoon chili powder
- 1 teaspoon cumin
- ½ teaspoon chipotle powder, or to taste
- ¼ – ½ teaspoon cinnamon, start small
- 1 small (1 ½ – 2lb.) butternut squash (about 4 – 5 cups), peeled, seeded & diced
- 2 red bell peppers, cored, seeded and diced
- 2 cans (15 oz) black beans, drained and rinsed, or 3 cups home cooked black beans
- 1 can (15 oz) fire roasted diced tomatoes + juice
- 2 cups water or vegetable broth
- 2 – 3 teaspoons cocoa powder or 1 oz of dark chocolate, optional
- Himalayan salt, to taste

INSTRUCTIONS

1. Stovetop: In a large 5 – 6 quart pot, heat oil/water over medium high heat, saute the onion for 5 – 7 minutes. Add the spices, saute for 1 minute more. Add the butternut squash, bell peppers, beans, tomatoes and vegetable broth and optional cocoa, bring to a boil, reduce heat, cover, and simmer for about 45 minutes. Will be done when the butternut squash is tender. Taste for flavor. Chili will thick upon cooling.

2. Slow Cooker: Place ingredients into your slow-cooker, finishing with the vegetable broth and give a good stir. Cover and cook on low for 6 – 8 hours, or on high for 3 – 4 hours. Taste, and season with additional salt and pepper or seasonings as needed.

3. Serve with garnish of choice. Pairs great with my favorite vegan cornbread or jalapeno cornbread muffins!

NUTRTION FACTS

Calories: 231kcal | Carbohydrates: 38g | Protein: 10g | Fat: 5g | Sodium: 898mg | Potassium: 816mg | Fiber: 10g | Sugar: 9g | Vitamin A: 4870IU | Vitamin C: 50.4mg | Calcium: 96mg | Iron: 4.4mg

CREAMY BUTTERNUT SQUASH PASTA SAUCE

Butternut squash pasta sauce is a perfect fall sauce for your favorite pasta or ravioli! Easy to make with simple ingredients and ready in about 30 minutes for a quick and easy weeknight meal.

Prep Time: 10 min Cook Time: 20 min Total Time: 30 minutes

Yield: Serves 4 – 6

INGREDIENTS

- 1 tablespoon olive oil or ¼ cup water/broth (for water sauté)

- 1 large shallot, diced

- 2 cloves garlic, minced (or 1 tsp. garlic powder)

- 1 small butternut squash (about 6 cups), diced

- 6 – 7 large sage leaves (about 2 – 3 tablespoons), chopped or 1 tablespoon dried

- ¼ – ½ teaspoon red pepper flakes, optional

- ⅛ tea spoon nutmeg

- 1 ½ cups vegetable broth

- ½ – 1 cup unsweetened almond milk or Vegan Cream, plus more as needed

- 1 cup cooked cannellini or great northern beans, optional

- Mineral salt & fresh cracked pepper, to taste

- 12 – 16 oz pasta of choice

INSTRUCTIONS

1. Pasta: Cook pasta of choice according to package directions, set aside.

2. Cube Squash: Slice off the very top and bottom, discard. Using a vegetable peeler, remove the hard outer skin. Cut the butternut squash in half, remove seeds and cut the squash into ½" cubes (the smaller the cubes are the quicker they will cook).

3. Cook: In a large pot, heat oil over medium heat, add shallots and sauté for 4 minutes or until softened. Add butternut squash, garlic, and herbs, cook another 4 minutes stirring occasionally. Add broth, bring to a boil, cover, and reduce heat to low and cook, occasionally stirring, until squash is softened, about 8 – 10 minutes. Add milk and optional beans to the pot.

4. Puree: Using an immersion blender or food processor/blender, blend until smooth or desired consistency (a little chunky is ok). If using a food processor or blender you may need to do it in two batches. Taste for seasoning. Add back to the pot and heat before serving if necessary.

5. Serve: To serve, add a little sauce to the bottom of your dish, and use the back of a spoon to spread the

sauce outward a bit making a circular or zigzag motion. Place pasta on top and cover with more sauce, gently toss to coat if you like (if you prefer, toss your pasta and sauce together in the pot and then serve). Top with optional toppings and fresh cracked pepper.

NUTRITION FACTS:

Cholesterol 5mg2% Sodium 487mg20% Potassium 344mg10% Carbohydrates 38g13%

Fiber 4g16% Sugar 2g2% Protein 9g18%

EASY LEMON ROSEMARY WHITE BEAN SOUP

Soothing and wholesome, this hearty white bean soup with lemon, herbs and veggies is healthy, full of flavor and a soup you'll want to make again and again! Quick and easy recipe, ready in 30 minutes.

Prep Time: 5 minutes

Cooking Time: 20 minutes

Total Time: 25 minutes

Yield: Serves 4 - 6

INGREDIENTS

- 2 tablespoons olive oil or ¼ cup water

- 1 small onion, diced

- large carrots, sliced or diced

- 2 stalks celery, sliced

- 2 cloves garlic, minced

- ½ teaspoon EACH dried thyme + rosemary
- cans (15oz) white beans (cannellini, great northern or chickpeas), drained and rinsed
- 5 cups low sodium vegetable broth
- 2 tablespoon tahini
- 1 – 2 lemons, juice of 1
- Salt + pepper
- Freshly chopped parsley, to serve

INSTRUCTIONS

1. Sauté: In a large pot, heat oil or water over medium heat, add onion, carrots, and celery, sauté for 7 minutes. Add garlic, thyme and rosemary and cook 1 minute more.

2. Simmer: Add the white beans, vegetable broth, tahini, and salt + pepper, give a good stir, bring to a boil, reduce heat to low, cover askew, and let simmer for 10 minutes, stirring occasionally.

3. Add lemon: Remove from heat, add lemon juice and let cool a bit before serving. The broth will thicken upon standing. Season with more salt, pepper or herbs as desired.

NUTRITION FACTS:

- Cholesterol 0mg   0% Sodium 357.6mg 16% Total Carbohydrate 56.3g 20%
- Dietary Fiber 17.4g 62%   Sugars   5.7g   Protein 19.4g39%

HOT SAUCE

Prep Time: 10 min

Cooking Time: 40 min

INGREDIENTS

- heads romaine lettuce, chopped
- 1 avocado, sliced (optional)
- Almond Parmesan
- Chickpea Croutons
- 1 can (15oz) chickpeas (garbanzo beans), drained and rinsed
- 1 tablespoon olive oil
- ¾ teaspoon garlic powder
- Generous pinch mineral salt
- Caesar Dressing
- ¾ cup raw cashews
- ½ cup water
- 2 garlic cloves
- 2 teaspoons capers
- 1 tablespoon vegan Worcester shire
- 2 teaspoons dijon mustard
- Juice of 1 medium lemon or 1 teaspoon apple cider vinegar
- Generous pinch of mineral salt & fresh cracked pepper

INSTRUCTIONS

1. Preheat oven to 400 degrees F. Line a rimmed baking sheet with parchment paper or Silpat.

2. Chickpea Croutons: Place rinsed chickpeas between a clean dish cloth, and gently rub them to dry, removing any of the loose skins. Place chickpeas on a prepared baking sheet, drizzle with oil and toss to coat, sprinkle with garlic powder and salt. Arrange chickpeas in a single layer, and garlic cloves (from the dressing), and bake for 40 – 45 minutes, stirring every 10 minutes or so. Remove the garlic if they seem to be getting too baked (especially if they are on the smaller side). Once done, set aside.

3. Caesar Salad Dressing: Soak the cashew in hot water (not boiling) for 5 minutes, drain. In a high speed or personal blender, add the cashews, water, roasted garlic cloves, capers, Worcestershire, dijon, lemon juice, salt & pepper, blend until creamy smooth. Makes a cup.

4. Assemble Caesar Salad: Place the chopped romaine in a large mixing bowl, add as much or as little of the dressing as you like, you may have some leftover, and give a good toss. Top with chickpea croutons, avocado, and a sprinkle of Almond Parmesan.

NUTRITION FACTS:

Calories: 0 Fat: 0g Sodium: 170mg

Carbohydrates: 0g Fiber: 0g Protein: 0g

SHRIMP SCAMPI

YIELD: 4 Servings

- PER SERVING: 1 Leanest, 3 Green, 2 Healthy Fat, 2½ Condiment.

- Total Time: 35 Minutes

INGREDIENTS

- 1 small to medium-sized spaghetti squash

- 2½ Tbsp olive oil

- 1 clove garlic, minced

- 1¾ lbs cooked, peeled, and deveined shrimp

- 1 cup cherry tomatoes, halved

- ½ tsp crushed red pepper flakes

- 1 tsp lemon juice

- 1 Tbsp dried parsley

- ½ tsp onion powder

- ¼ tsp salt

- ¼ tsp ground pepper

- ¼ cup shredded Parmesan cheese

DIRECTIONS

1. Cut squash in half, and remove seeds. Place in both halves in a microwave-safe bowl with an inch of water. Microwave for 10 to 12 minutes, or until tender (microwave time will vary based on exact size of squash and power of microwave).

2. Allow squash to cool before handling. Use a fork to scrape out flesh into spaghetti-like strands. Measure out 5 cups; save extra for another meal.

3. Heat a large skillet over medium-high heat. Add olive oil and swirl to the coat pan. Sauté the garlic until fragrant, about one minute.

4. Add the shrimp, tomatoes, crushed red pepper flakes, lemon juice, parsley, onion powder, salt, and pepper; cook for 3 to 4 minutes. Add the spaghetti squash, and continue to cook until heated through. Remove from heat, and sprinkle parmesan cheese on top.

NUTRITION FACTS:

Total Fat 30.5g 39% Tot. Carb. 32.6g Sat. Fat 11.9g59% Dietary Fiber 0.2g

Trans Fat 2.3g Sugars 2g Cholesterol 78.1mg 26% Protein 13.1g

BERRY + SPINACH QUINOA SALAD

Prep Time: 5 min

Cooking Time: 25 min

Yield: Serves 4

INGREDIENTS

- 1 cup dried quinoa, rinsed
- 1 ¾ cup water
- 5 oz. baby spinach (about 5 cups)
- 1 cup blueberries
- 1 cup strawberries, sliced
- 1 cup blackberries
- ⅓ Cup slivered almonds

- Sliced avocado, optional
- Citrus Dressing
- ⅓ cup orange juice
- 2 teaspoons apple cider vinegar
- 2 teaspoons Dijon
- 2 teaspoons pure maple syrup
- Salt + pepper, to taste

INSTRUCTIONS

1. Quinoa: In a small pot, add quinoa and water, bring to a boil, cover, reduce heat to low and simmer for 15 minutes. Remove lid and let rest for 10 minutes, fluff with a fork. In a small bowl, combine the dressing ingredients and mix well.

2. Dressing: In a small bowl, whisk together the ingredients for the citrus dressing. Set aside until ready to serve.

3. Salad: In a large bowl add the spinach, quinoa, blueberries, strawberries and slivered almonds. Pour dressing over the top and toss well to coat. Serve at room temperature or chilled in individual bowls with optional sliced avocado and a little extra slivered almonds on top.

NUTRITION FACTS:

Serving size: 1 salad Calories: 320 Fat: 18g Saturated fat: 3g Carbohydrates: 21g Sodium: 51mg Fiber: 9g Protein: 21g Cholesterol: 47mg

HEALTHY RAINBOW SALAD

Light, bright and delicious, this healthy Asian inspired Rainbow Salad is for those days when you're feeling the need to eat lighter or getting in that daily raw meal! Sugar free and oil free

Prep Time: 10 min

Cooking Time: 5 min

Yield: Serves 4

INGREDIENTS

- 1 head romaine, sliced
- 1 small head savoy cabbage, or ½ head large, sliced
- ¼ head red cabbage, sliced

- 1 red bell pepper, sliced
- 1 yellow bell pepper, sliced

- 2 scallions, sliced
- ½ cup cilantro, roughly chopped

TO SERVE

- Mango dressing, use full recipe
- 1 avocado, sliced
- Black sesame seeds
- Slivered almonds

INSTRUCTIONS

1. Salad: Add romaine and cabbage to a large bowl. Add the bell peppers, scallions, and cilantro over the greens. Toss to mix.

2. Serve: Serve in individual dishes, top with diced avocado and spicy mango dressing. Add a sprinkle of black sesame seeds and slivered almonds over the top. If eating this as a monster salad, simply enjoy straight from the large bowl.

3. Makes one very large salad or four smaller salads.

NUTRITION FACTS:

- Calories: 39 Protein: 1.3 g Carbohydrate: 8.4 g Sugar: 5.9 g Fat: 0.4 g

- Calories from fat: 9.2% Fiber: 1.3 g Sodium: 87 mg

VEGAN MINESTRONE SOUP

Loaded with veggies, beans and pasta, this Vegan Minestrone Soup is healthy, comforting and so easy to make in one pot and ready in about 30 minutes!

Prep Time: 5 min

Cooking Time: 25 min

Yield: Serves 4 – 6

INGREDIENTS

- 1 tablespoon olive oil or ¼ cup water for water sauté

- 1 medium onion, diced

- 2 medium carrots, diced2 celery ribs, diced

- 3 – 4 cloves garlic, minced 1 zucchini, cut into half moons

- ⅓ Pound green beans (about 1 ½ cup), cut into 1 inch pieces

- 1 can (14oz) kidney beans, drained and rinsed

- 1 can (14oz) chickpeas (garbanzo beans), drained and rinsed

- 1 can (28oz) diced tomatoes, with juices

- 2 teaspoons Italian seasoning blendPinch of red pepper flakes

- 2 – 3 bay leaves

- 1 cup small pasta (mini penne, rotini) 4 cups vegetable broth

- 2 – 4 cups water2 handfuls fresh spinach

- Mineral salt & pepper to tasteLemon juice

- Fresh parsley, chopped

INSTRUCTIONS

1. Sauté: In a large dutch oven or pot, add the oil or water and sauté the onion, carrot and celery for 5 minutes. Alternately, you can skip sautéing and add all the ingredients, except for the spinach, to a large pot, bring to a boil and continue with the recipe as written. This makes for one less step!

2. Cook: Add remaining ingredients, except the spinach, bring to a boil, cover askew, reduce heat to low and simmer at a gentle boil for 20 – 25 minutes, stirring occasionally. Soup is done when veggies are tender and pasta is cooked. Add more broth or water as needed.

3. Add spinach: Five minutes before the soup is done, add the spinach and stir to mix.

4. Let soup cool a few minutes and serve with a squeeze of lemon and chopped parsley on top. Pairs will come with homemade Vegan Cornbread, crusty Artisan Bread or soft and chewy Vegan Naan for soaking up the juices.

NUTRITION FACTS:

Calories: 203 Protein: 9 g Carbohydrates: 41 g Sugar: 7 g Fat: 1 g Calories from Fat: 6% Fiber: 7 g Sodium: 396 mg

.

EASY LEMON ROSEMARY WHITE BEAN SOUP

Easy White Bean Soup with soothing lemon, veggies, rosemary, thyme and tahini is healthy and easy to make using everyday ingredients that you probably already have on hand! It's full of nutrition, flavor and is amazingly delicious!

This vegan white bean soup is so full of deliciousness. Plus, it's well-balanced, full of healthy protein & fiber, and can be made oil-free! The hearty texture, subtle combination of flavors and yummy creaminess from the tahini will leave you wanting more. It's a perfect pantry friendly soup that has it all.

INGREDIENTS

- Onion, carrots, celery and garlic are sautéed, simmered with white beans, herbs and tahini creating a wholesome and healthy soup that's perfect for a satisfying vegan lunch, dinner or meal prep idea.

- White beans – cannellini or great northern beans are preferred, but chickpeas will work too. Even a combo is great!

- Onion – brown or white

- Carrots – I used 3 large carrots for extra heartiness

- Celery – feel free to add in a few celery leaves as well

- Garlic – sub with 1 teaspoon garlic paste or garlic powder

- Thyme + rosemary – dried is fine, but fresh is great too

- Tahini – adds a nice flavor and creaminess, sub with cashew butter (can be optional)

- Vegetable broth – ½ teaspoon Better than Bouillon Veg Base with water.

- Lemon – Lemon for the soup and the other for garnish and squeezing into serving bowl.

- Salt + pepper – to taste

INSTRUCTIONS

1. In a large pot, heat oil or water over medium heat, add onion, carrots, and celery, saute for 7 minutes.

2. Add garlic, thyme and rosemary and cook 1 minute more.

3. Add the white beans, vegetable broth, and salt + pepper.

4. Give a good stir, add the tahini, bring to a boil, reduce heat to low, cover askew, and let simmer for 10 minutes, stirring occasionally.

5. Remove from heat, add lemon juice and let cool a bit before serving (shown below). The broth will thicken upon standing—season with more salt, pepper or herbs as desired.

6. Add a few handfuls of spinach at the end of cooking, letting it wilt and soften, for extra color and nutrition.

7. The soup will thicken as it cools, that's if you can wait that long!

8. To thicken the soup even more, or if not using tahini, mash some of the beans with the back of a spoon to add creaminess.

9. Serve with homemade Artisan Bread, soft and chewy Vegan Naan or gluten-free Socca flatbread to soak up the juices.

NUTRITION FACTS:

- Total Fat 5.2g 7% Saturated Fat 0.9g Cholesterol 0mg 0% Sodium 357.6mg 16%

- Total Carbohydrate 56.3g 20% Dietary Fiber 17.4g 62% Sugars 5.7g Protein 19.4g 39%

ROASTED BUTTERNUT SQUASH SALAD

Roasted Butternut Squash Salad with tender winter squash, cranberries, pepitas, fresh greens, and tossed with simple shallot vinaigrette is perfect for entertainment.

Whether entertaining a crowd or craving an easy fall salad for yourself, this roasted butternut squash salad is perfect! It's healthy, easy to make and is perfect for the holiday or potluck table, as well as a simple lunch, dinner or meal prep idea.

INGREDIENTS

- Butternut Squash.

- Use small butternut squash, 1 ½ lb. or so.

- Oil (any neutral oil)

- Pure Maple Syrup- Adds a hint of maple flavor when roasting the butternut squash.

- Dried Cranberries- Add the cranberries with the butternut squash for the last 5 minutes of cooking to warm them up a bit. Feel free to use raisins or fresh pomegranate seeds in place of cranberries.

- Pepitas- Use pecans, walnuts or almonds in place of the pumpkin seeds (preferably).

- Shallots- Smaller than an onion, shallots have a mild onion flavor with a hint of garlic. It will be added to the dressing for a shallot vinaigrette.

- Apple Cider Vinegar- Use white wine or champagne vinegar.

- Dijon

- Salt & Pepper

- Leafy Greens- (kale, spinach, arugula)

INSTRUCTIONS

1. Roast the butternut squash. Prep the butternut squash and toss with olive oil, maple syrup, salt & pepper, spread on a rimmed baking sheet and bake for 30 minutes at 425 degrees.

2. Dressing: This salad is paired with a simple shallot vinaigrette which I just love. Simply mix the ingredients together and let rest while the squash is roasting. To make an oil free vinaigrette for this salad,

use apple juice or apple cider in place of the oil. Feel free to warm your dressing just before serving, or keep it near a warm spot by the stove until ready to serve. This salad would also be great with a sweeter dressing like this Maple Dijon Dressing (just double the recipe).

3. Assemble the salad. Add your leafy greens to a large platter or serving bow.

4. Top with butternut squash, sprinkle of cranberries and pepitas.

5. Drizzle the dressing overtop, season with more salt and pepper to taste.

NUTRITION FACTS:

Per Serving: 299 calories; fat 14g; saturated fat 2g; mono fat 8g; poly fat 3g; Protein 8g; carbohydrates 42g; fiber 8g; Iron 3mg; sodium 325mg; calcium 237mg.

WARM CAPER + BEET SALAD

Serves: 4-6

Time: 35 minutes (5 minutes prep time, 30 minutes cook time)

Fresh beets are a neglected vegetable, probably because people aren't sure how to cook them. In the pressure cooker, it's very easy, and these bright purple nutrition bombs go really well with ingredients like garlic, rice wine vinegar, and capers. It's nice to have a salad option that doesn't involve greens.

INGREDIENTS

- medium-sized beets

- 1 cup water

- 2 tablespoons rice wine vinegar

- 1 garlic clove

- 2 tablespoons capers

- 1 tablespoon of chopped parsley

- 1 tablespoon olive oil

- ½ teaspoon salt

- ½ teaspoon black pepper

DIRECTIONS

1. Pour one cup of water into your pressure cooker and lower in the steamer basket

2. Clean and trim the beets

3. Put beets in the steamer basket

4. Close and seal the lid

5. Select "manual" and cook on high pressure for 25 minutes

6. While that cooks, make the dressing by shaking chopped garlic, parsley, oil, salt, pepper, and capers in a jar.

7. When time is up, hit "cancel" and carefully quick-release the pressure

8. Beets should be soft enough to pierce with a fork

9. Run the beets under cold water and remove the skins

10. Slice beets and serve with rice wine vinegar and jar dressing.

NUTRITION FACTS

- Total calories: 43.1
- Protein: .7
- Carbs: 5.4
- Fiber: .8 Fat: 2.4

SOUTHWESTERN SALAD

Southwestern Salad is a fresh and colorful, well-rounded salad that's cool, crisp and full of zesty Tex-Mex flavor!

Prep Time: 15 min Cook Time: 10 Total Time: 25 minutes

Yield: Serves 2 - 3 1x

INGREDIENTS

- 2 heads romaine lettuce, chopped
- 1 can (15 oz) black beans, drained and rinsed or 1 ½ cups cooked
- 2 corn off the cob (about 1 – 1 ¼ cups), canned (drained) or frozen (thawed) ok too
- Handful grape tomatoes, halved
- Handful mini sweet peppers, sliced
- ½ cup onion (sliced green onion or diced red onion), optional
- 1 avocado, sliced
- Lime wedges, to serve
- Cilantro sprigs, to serve
- Salt + pepper, to taste

- 1 batch Hatch Chile Dressing, or see notes for Cilantro-Lime Vinaigrette

INSTRUCTIONS

1. Dressing: Make the dressing, set it aside on the counter or refrigerate.

2. Salad: Prep the ingredients. In individual serving bowls, add the romaine, top with black beans, corn, tomatoes, mini peppers, cilantro, and avocado. Drizzle with dressing. Top with salt and pepper to taste.

NUTRITION FACTS:

- Total Fat 6.3ggrams 8%Saturated Fat 1.5ggrams

- Trans Fat 0.1ggrams 2%Cholesterol 5.7mgmilligrams 14%Sodium 343mgmilligrams

- 6%Potassium 215mgmilligrams 5%Total Carbohydrates 14ggrams

- 14%Dietary Fiber 3.5ggrams Sugars 2.2ggrams Protein 4.1g

THAI CRUNCH SALAD + CITRUS PEANUT DRESSING

Top down view of a large serving bowl with mixed Thai crunch salad and stainless steel Salad utensils with black handles

Prep Time: 15 min Total Time: 15 min

Yield: Serves 2 - 3 1x

INGREDIENTS

- 2 ½ cups English cucumbers, thinly sliced and halved or quartered
- 1 cup carrots, thinly sliced
- 1 red bell pepper, julienned
- 2 scallions, thinly sliced
- 1 small head Napa cabbage (about 2 – 3 cups), sliced
- ¼ head of red cabbage, sliced
- Handful peanuts or cashews, for garnish
- Handful cilantro, for garnish (optional)
- Red pepper flakes, for garnish (optional)
- Citrus Peanut Dressing:
- tablespoons orange juice, lime juice or lemon juice, + more as needed
- tablespoons raw or natural peanut butter (almond or cashew butter is great too)
- 1 tablespoon tamari, coconut aminos or soy sauce
- 1 tablespoon pure maple syrup
- 1 garlic clove, grated
- ½ teaspoon fresh ginger, grated
- Pinch of red pepper flakes or ½ teaspoon sriracha hot sauce (optional)

INSTRUCTIONS

1. **Dressing:** In a small bowl, whisk together the ingredients for the peanut citrus dressing, set aside

allowing the flavors to come together. Then before adding the dressing to the salad, taste for flavor adding anything extra you might like. For a thinner dressing add 1 or 2 tablespoons citrus juice or water. To make it thicker add a tad bit more nut butter.

2. **Assemble:** Prepare your salad ingredients. Check your dressing for flavor. In a large bowl the napa and red cabbage, scallions, red bell pepper, cucumber, carrots and peanuts or cashews, pour the dressing over the top the salad and toss well to coat.

NUTRITION FACTS

- Fat 34g52% Saturated Fat 13g65% Cholesterol 9mg3% Sodium 1239mg52%

- Potassium 694mg20% Carbohydrates 31g10% Fiber 6g24% Sugar 20g22%

- Protein 16g32%

LEMON CHICKPEA ORZO SOUP (VEGAN AVGOLEMONO)

Lemon Chickpea Orzo Soup (aka Greek vegan avgolemono soup) features soothing citrus, chickpeas, orzo, refreshing dill and fresh baby greens with tahini for added creaminess!

INGREDIENTS

- Olive oil – use water for oil free

- Onion

- Carrots

- Garlic

- Vegetable broth – or combo of water and veg broth

- Orzo – whole wheat pref

- Chickpeas – aka garbanzo beans

- Tahini – store bought or make homemade Tahini

- Lemon juice (about 3 – 4 large lemons)

- Baby kale or spinach

- Dill – use fresh, as much as you like

- Salt + pepper – lemon-pepper would be great too!

INSTRUCTIONS

1. Sauté the onion and carrot, sauté for about 5 – 7 minutes, add the garlic and sauté for 1 minute more.

2. Simmer with chickpeas and orzo. Add the broth or water, bring to a boil, add the orzo and chickpeas, reduce heat to medium-low and cook at a gentle boil for 7 – 8 minutes.

3. Add brightness + creaminess. Once done, turn the heat off and stir in the tahini and lemon juice.

4. Add leafy greens. Add the baby kale or spinach, give a good stir, greens will soften and wilt within a few minutes.

5. Stir in herbs + season. Add as much dill as you like, and season well with salt & pepper.

6. Top down view of healthy chickpea lemon orzo soup in a large pot.

NUTRITION FACTS:

- Total Fat 12.3g 16% Saturated Fat 1.7g   Cholesterol 0mg   0%

- Sodium 713.6mg   31% Total Carbohydrate 42.9g 16% Dietary Fiber 9.6g   34%

- Sugars 9.6g   Protein 12.3g   25%

HEARTY CHICKPEA NOODLE SOUP (VEGAN)

Forget chicken noodle soup, this vegan Chickpea Noodle Soup recipe is loaded with veggies, protein rich chickpeas, hearty pasta & flavorful herbs, and ready in 30 minutes!

INGREDIENTS

- Veggies – The veggies are the usual staples of carrots, celery and onion. This flavorful mirepoix is all you really need, but I don't doubt a few handfuls of fresh baby spinach at the end of cooking would be nice too!

- Pasta – Use whole grain or regular pasta. I used rotini, but any bite sized pasta will be great. See below for the GF option.

- Chickpeas – Not much to say about this one, except I ♡ chickpeas!

- Herbs – Herbs can be versatile using what you have on hand. I've used a combination of dried basil, oregano and thyme, but really any one or two of these will be fine. The bay leaves are subtle, you can do without those if needed. Finally, the parsley at the end adds fresh, bright flavors and is SO good!

- Liquids – This chickpea noodle soup calls for 10 – 12 cups of liquids, which can be water, vegetable broth or combo of the two. I used water with about 1 teaspoon of Better

NUTRITION FACTS:

- Total Fat 3.1g4% Saturated Fat 0.4g Cholesterol 0mg 0%

- Sodium 411.2mg   18% Total Carbohydrate 69.5g 25%

- Dietary Fiber 9g   32% Sugars 8.5g   Protein 14.4g 29%

LEMONY KALE & WHITE BEAN SOUP

You're going to love how simple this recipe is, using everyday accessible ingredients. This kale and white bean soup takes 30 minutes to make and only one pot. It's filled with healthy, whole foods to keep you happy and nourished.

Prep Time: 10 min Cook Time: 30 min Total Time: 40 minutes

Yield: Serves 4 - 6 1x

INGREDIENTS

- 1 tablespoon olive oil or ½ cup water for water sauté

- 2 medium leeks (about 3 – 4 cups), thinly sliced (white & pale green parts only)

- 2 large carrots (about 1 cup), diced

- 2 celery stalks (about 1 cup), diced

- 2 garlic cloves, minced

- 1 teaspoon dried oregano, rosemary or thyme or 2 teaspoons fresh chopped

- Pinch of red pepper flakes

- 6 – 7 cups low-sodium vegetable broth or combo of water & broth

- 2 cans (15 oz) cannellini beans, drained and rinsed or 3 cups cooked

- 1 bunch kale (marinate or curly), middle stem removed and julienned

- 2 – 3 lemons, juice of

- Mineral salt & fresh cracked pepper to taste

- Chopped parsley, to serve

INSTRUCTIONS

1. In a large pot or dutch oven, heat oil or water over medium heat, add leeks, carrots, celery, and sauté for about 5 – 7 minutes (leeks should be softened and wilted). Add garlic and herbs & red pepper flakes, sauté 1 minute more or until fragrant.

2. Boil & Simmer: Add liquids and beans, bring to a slight boil, add kale, turn down heat to low and cook until kale softens and wilts, about 5 minutes. Add lemon juice and salt & pepper to taste. Add extra water/broth as needed.

3. Serve with a sprinkle of parsley and a squeeze of lemon. A light dusting of Almond Parmesan would be a nice touch too. Pair with your favorite crusty bread or naan bread to soak up the juices.

NUTRITION FACTS:

- Calories: 574kcal Carbohydrates: 106g Protein: 22g Fat: 16g Sodium: 177mg

- Fiber: 23g Sugar: 9g Calcium: 110mg Iron: 2.2mg

DESSERTS

CRANBERRY ALMOND ENERGY BITES (NO BAKE)

Naturally sweetened and so easy to make, no bake Cranberry Energy Bites with almonds, cranberries and oats are a healthy, wholesome treat perfect for snacking or dessert!

Prep Time: 30 min Total Time: 30 minutes

Yield: Makes 20

INGREDIENTS

- 1 cup raw almonds

- 1 cup dried cranberries

- 1 cup old fashioned oats

- ½ cup shredded coconut

- ½ cup pure maple syrup or 1 cup pitted Medjool dates (11 – 12), chopped

- 1 teaspoon vanilla

- Pinch of salt

INSTRUCTIONS

1. **Blend:** Add ingredients to the bowl of a food processor and blend until mixed well and crumbly, stopping to scrape down the sides as needed.

2. **Chill:** Place the mixture in the refrigerator for about 20 minutes to let it stiffen up a bit.

3. **Scoop and roll:** Using a 1 tablespoon measuring spoon, scoop up rounded mounds and roll into 1 inch balls.

4. Add the finishing touch. For a more finished look and to keep the dough from sticking to your fingers, roll the energy bites in shredded coconut or almond flour.

NUTRITION FACTS

- Amount Per Serving: CALORIES: 99 TOTAL FAT: 6Gs ATURATED FAT: 1g

- TRANS FAT:0g UNSATURATED FAT: 4g CHOLESTEROL: 2mg SODIUM: 36mg

- CARBOHYDRATES: 12g FIBER: 2g SUGAR: 8g PROTEIN: 2g

CRISPY ROASTED CHICKPEAS RECIPE

Packed with protein and fiber, oven roasted chickpeas make a great snack or crispy addition to salads, soups and meal bowls.

Prep Time: 10 min Cook Time: 40 min Total Time: 50 minutes

Yield: Serves 3

INGREDIENTS

- 1 can (15oz) chickpeas (garbanzo beans) or 1 ½ cups fresh cooked

- 1 – 2 teaspoons olive oil

- 1 teaspoon flavor seasoning – garlic salt or lemon-pepper

- Generous pinch of salt

INSTRUCTIONS

- Preheat the oven to 400 degrees F.

- Prep: If you're using canned chickpeas, place them in a colander and rinse them under cool running water.

- Dry: Fold a large dish towel or flour sack in half, placing the chickpeas between. With your hands laid flat, roll the chickpeas using the palm of your hand and extended fingers to move the garbanzo beans around. Try to remove as much moisture as you can.

- Remove loose skins: Once dry, pick away any skins that have noticeably become detached or loosened by gently pinching the chickpeas between your thumb and forefinger. Repeat rolling the chickpeas one more time for good measure.

- Oil & Season: Spread the chickpeas onto a rimmed baking sheet lined with parchment paper or Silpat (affiliate links), lightly greased is ok. Drizzle with a teaspoon or two of olive oil, add seasoning and mix well to coat. Arrange the chickpeas across the baking sheet in a single layer.

- Roast: Bake for 40 – 45 minutes, stirring every 10 minutes or so. Once done let cool a bit before using or storing.

NUTRITION FACT:

Serving Size: 1/4 Cup Per Serving: 100 calories; protein 6g; carbohydrates 17g; dietary fiber 5g; sugars 3g; fat 1.5g; sodium 170mg.

2-MINUTE STEAMED ASPARAGUS

Serves: 3-4

Time: 2 minutes

Get fresh asparagus when it's in season from February through June, and steam up a batch in your pressure cooker in just two minutes. Asparagus is super healthy, but it's accessible to under or overcooks it. Luckily, the pressure cooker takes care of that, so you get perfectly steamed veggies every time.

INGREDIENTS

- 1 lb. trimmed asparagus
- 1 cup of water
- 2 tablespoons olive oil
- 1 tablespoon of minced onion
- Sea salt and pepper to taste
- Squeeze of fresh lemon

DIRECTIONS

1. Pour water into your pressure cooker and lower in the steamer basket
2. Put the asparagus in the basket
3. Drizzle on a little olive oil and onion

4. Close and seal the lid

5. Select "steam" and adjust the time to 2 minutes

6. When time is up, hit "cancel" and quick-release the pressure

7. Serve with salt, pepper, and a squeeze of lemon juice.

NUTRITION FACTS (1/4 Recipe):

- Total calories: 84

- Protein: 3g

- Carbs: 5g

- Fiber: 4g

- Fat: 0g

STEAMED ARTICHOKES

Serves: 6

Time: 33 minutes (10 minutes prep time, 5 minutes cook time, 15 minutes dry time, 3 minutes fry time).

Artichokes are one of the healthiest veggies out there, but their intimidating hard bodies put a lot of people off. The prep is worth the result, especially when you can steam the artichokes to perfection in your pressure cooker. After cooking, you finish them off with a little frying in a separate skillet.

INGREDIENTS

- 6 long, narrow artichokes

- smashed garlic cloves

- 2 cups water

- 1-2 cups of olive oil

- Juice of 1 lemon

- 1 sliced lemon

- 1 tablespoon whole peppercorns

DIRECTIONS

1. Pour 2 cups of water, lemon juice, lemon slices, and peppercorns into your pressure cooker

2. Prep artichokes by tearing off the tough leaves on the outside, peeling the stem, cutting off the end of the stem, and cutting the top half off of the leaves horizontally, so you end up with what looks like a hat

3. Pry open the leaves and take out the hairy, hard part to access the heart, leaving the dotty part where the hairy part was attached

4. Open the leaves up a bit more and dip in the pressure cooker, head down, and swirl around before putting them in the steamer basket

5. Put basket with artichokes in the pressure cooker, Close and seal lid.

6. Select "manual" and cook on high pressure for 5 minutes

7. When time is up, quick-release the pressure after hitting "cancel."

8. Shake the artichokes and put them in a strainer for 15 minutes to dry out

9. In a pan, heat up about 2 centimeters of oil and just fry the artichokes head down until their edges start to turn golden

10. Plate and dab with a paper towel to remove excess oil before serving.

NUTRITION FACTS

- Total calories: 40
- Protein: 1g
- Carbs: 3g
- Fiber: 9g
- Fat: 2g

CLASSIC HUMMUS (OIL FREE)

Serves: 6-8

Time: 28 minutes (18 minutes cook time, 10 minutes natural release)

A traditional Middle Eastern spread, hummus can be expensive when you get it in the store, and there are always listeria recalls going on. That's not very delicious. Thankfully, you can make your own hummus in the pressure cooker very easily, and season it to your liking, whether you're a garlic lover and prefer it to be a bit more-mild. Remember - you have to soak dry chickpeas overnight.

INGREDIENTS

- 6 cups water
- 1 cup soaked chickpeas
- 3-4 crushed garlic cloves
- 1 bay leaf
- ¼ cup chopped parsley
- 2 tablespoons tahini
- 1 juiced lemon

- ½ teaspoon salt

- ¼ teaspoon cumin

- Dash of paprika

DIRECTIONS

1. Soak your chickpeas overnight in water

2. When you're ready to make the hummus, rinse them and put them in the pressure cooker

3. Pour in 6 cups of water

4. Toss in the bay leaf and garlic cloves

5. Close and seal the lid

6. Select "manual," and cook for 18 minutes on high pressure

7. When the beeper goes off, hit "cancel" and wait for the pressure to come down on its own

8. When the cooker is safe to open, drain the chickpeas, but save all the cooking liquid

9. Remove the bay leaf before pureeing the chickpeas

10. Add tahini, lemon juice, cumin, and ½ cup of cooking liquid to start

11. Keep pureeing, and if the mixture isn't creamy enough, keep adding ½ cup of liquid at a time

12. When it's the right level of creaminess, salt, and puree once more

13. Serve with a sprinkle of paprika and fresh chopped parsley!

NUTRITION FACTS

- Total calories: 109
- Protein: 4.1g
- Carbs: 3.5g
- Fiber: 3.3g
- Fat: 3.8g

EASY VEGAN STRAWBERRY SHORTCAKE

Vegan Strawberry Shortcake with fluffy and tender, sweet biscuits filled with juicy strawberries and coconut whipped cream is a perfect summer treat and so easy to make!

Prep Time: 15 min Cook Time: 10 min Total Time: 25 minutes

Yield: 12 Servings

INGREDIENTS

- Strawberries + Coconut Whipped Cream
- 1 lb. fresh strawberries, tops removed and chopped
- 2 teaspoons organic pure cane sugar
- Coconut whip cream
- Shortcake Biscuits
- 1 cup unsweetened almond milk (use your favorite non-dairy milk)
- Juice of 1 lemon or 2 teaspoons apple cider vinegar

- cups flour (unbleached all-purpose, or half mix with spelled or white whole wheat)

- ¼ cup organic pure cane sugar

- teaspoons baking powder

- ¼ teaspoon mineral salt

- ½ cup coconut oil, at room temperature or hard (cubed vegan butter is ok too)

INSTRUCTIONS

1. Preheat oven to 425 degrees F.

2. Vegan Buttermilk: Measure the milk and the juice of 1 lemon or apple cider vinegar, let rest for 5 – 10 minutes to curdle.

3. Strawberries: Place the strawberries in a medium bowl with 2 teaspoons pure cane sugar and combine. Set aside for at least 20 minutes. The longer they rest, the more juicer (more macerated) they will become.

Shortcakes:

1. Dry ingredients: In a large mixing bowl, combine the flour, sugar, baking powder and salt.

2. Cut the oil (or butter): Add the coconut oil and cut the oil into the flour using a fork or pastry blender. When done flour should be lumpy with little balls of flour.

3. Combine dry and wet: Pour the vegan buttermilk into the flour mixture and mix to combine. Don't overmix the dough, mix just until combined.

4. Flatten dough: Once the dough is formed, place it on a lightly floured flat surface. Using your hands, flatten and mold the dough into a circle shape about ½ inch thick (a rolling pin will work too).

5. Cut dough: Cut circles using a 3 inch cookie cutter (a glass is ok too). Dip the cutter in flour before each cut to keep it from sticking. Leftover dough can be reshaped and cut. You should get 12 shortcakes.

6. Prep for baking: Place the shortcakes on an UNGREASED baking sheet, or lined with a Silpat or parchment paper. Make sure the sides are touching each other, this will make them cling to one another, rising bigger and taller.

7. Garnish biscuits: Brush the tops with a little almond milk and sprinkle with pure cane sugar or turbinado. The sugar will give the shortcake tops a nice crunchy texture.

8. Bake: Place shortcakes in the oven and bake for 15 minutes. Let cool a few minutes before assembling your strawberry shortcakes.

9. Assemble shortcakes: To serve, slice shortcakes in half, top with strawberries and a generous dollop of vegan whipped cream.

10. Makes 12 strawberry shortcakes.

11. More recommendable is the unbleached all-purpose flour when making shortcakes. It yields the most tender and fluffiest biscuits. You could also try half all-purpose and half whole grain; just don't skimp on the oil or butter.

12. Tips for cutting biscuits:

13. To keep the dough from sticking to the cutter, keep a small bowl or plate of flour nearby and dip the cutter into the flour, shaking any loose flour away, before making cuts.

14. Don't twist the cutter when making cuts, it creates a seal and the biscuits won't rise as well.

NUTRITION FACTS

- Serving: 1bar Calories: 66kcal Carbohydrates: 31g Protein: 2g Fat: 1g Sodium: 85mg

- Potassium: 85mg Fiber: 2g Sugar: 2g Vitamin C: 23mg Calcium: 1mg Iron: 4mg

RAW CHOCOLATE AVOCADO PUDDING

Raw Chocolate Avocado Pudding with 3 flavor combinations, creating a deliciously healthy and dairy-free pudding that will rival any other!

Prep Time: 5 min Total Time: 5 min

Yield: Serves 2

Category: Snack, Dessert

INGREDIENTS

- SCALE

- Chocolate Avocado Pudding Base

- 1 large avocado (or 2 small), skin and seed removed

- 1 ripe banana, peeled

- 4 tablespoons cacao powder

- 4 tablespoons pure maple syrup, coconut nectar or date syrup

- 1 teaspoon vanilla extract

- ¼ teaspoon cinnamon, optional

- **Orange Chocolate Avocado Pudding**

- ½ cup fresh squeezed orange juice, + more as needed

- 1 teaspoon or so orange zest, optional

- **Chocolate Espresso Avocado Pudding**

- 1 teaspoon instant espresso powder

INSTRUCTIONS

1. In a blender, combine the base pudding ingredients (along with any one of the optional flavor combinations) and blend until creamy, stopping to scrape down the sides as needed. Add water, a few tablespoons at a time, as needed for desired consistency. Typically I use ½ cup of water, unless making the orange flavored. Taste for flavor and adjust accordingly.

2. Pudding can be served at room temp, but I find it's best when chilled in the refrigerator for a couple of hours.

3. Serve: Top with a dollop of whipped coconut cream and shaved dark chocolate, cacao nibs or carob chips.

4. Store: Leftovers can be stored in an airtight container in the refrigerator for 4 – 5 days. To freeze, store in Popsicle molds for best results, can be kept in the freezer for up to 2 months.

NOTES

Feel free to omit the banana, using an extra avocado in its place.

Nutritional values are estimates only. See our full nutrition disclosure here.

NUTRITION FACTS:

calories: 255kcal, carbohydrates: 25g, Protein: 4g, Fat: 17g, saturated fat: 2g, sodium: 50mg, potassium: 608mg, Fiber: 8g, sugar: 12g, vitamin a: 165iu, vitamin c: 10.1mg, calcium: 83mg, iron: 1.8mg

BEST VEGAN CHOCOLATE CHIP COOKIES

The best vegan chocolate chip cookie recipe with no funny ingredients and no chilling time! Just simple, straightforward, amazingly delicious chocolate chip cookies that bake up perfectly every single time!

Prep Time: 10 min

Cook Time: 10 min

Total Time: 20 minutes

Yield: Makes 24 cookies

INGREDIENTS

- ½ cup (113g) vegan butter (Miyoko's), at room temp
- ½ cup (85g) coconut sugar
- ¼ cup (43g) pure cane sugar
- tablespoons unsweetened cashew or almond milk
- 2 teaspoons vanilla extract
- 1 ½ cups flour (light spelled (148g), all-purpose (180g) or gluten free flour blend)
- ½ teaspoon baking soda
- ¼ teaspoon mineral salt

- 1 cup (175g) vegan chocolate chips (I used Enjoy Life)

INSTRUCTIONS

1. Preheat oven to 350 degrees F. Line a baking sheet with parchment paper or Silpat, or use a baking sheet as is, un-greased.

2. Cookie Dough: Combine flour, baking soda and salt in small bowl. Beat butter, coconut sugar and pure cane sugar in large mixing bowl until creamy. Add almond milk and vanilla extract, and beat until fluffy and creamy, about 1 – 2 minutes. Add ½ of the flour and mix to combine, add remaining flour and mix again. Stir in chocolate chips.

3. Scoop: Drop rounded 1 ½ – 2 tablespoons full of cookie dough onto a prepared baking sheet, keeping them about 2 inches apart.

4. Bake: Place in the oven and bake for 10 to 12 minutes (don't overbake). Cool on baking sheets for 2 minutes, move to wire racks to cool.

5. Makes 2 dozen cookies.

NOTES

1. Substitute the butter with room temp coconut oil. When using room temp coconut oil, make sure all other wet ingredients are at room temp as well, or the coconut oil will seize up and harden.

2. Optional Add-Ins: Add nuts such as chopped pecans, walnuts, or pistachios. Dried fruits like cherries or cranberries would be delicious.

3. Pull the butter out early so it has time to come to room temperature. It's important that the butter is softened, but not melted so it will cream well with the sugars.

4. Don't overcook the cookies. They will look tender and slightly underdone but will firm up as they cool.

5. If using all coconut sugar, your cookies will be darker in color. This will also happen if using a heavier flour such as whole wheat. For lighter cookies, use a mix of white and brown sugars, and all-purpose or light spelt flour.

NUTRITION FACTS:

1. Saturated Fat 14g70% Trans Fat g Cholesterol 0mg0% Sodium 450mg19%

2. Potassium 85mg2% Total Carbohydrates 50g17% Dietary Fiber 1g4% Sugars 21g Protein 4g8%

CHOCOLATE PEANUT BUTTER NO-BAKE COOKIES

Chocolate + peanut butter + oatmeal combination is a winning combination! This classic No Bake Cookies recipe is healthy and easy to make.

Prep Time: 10 min Total Time: 10 minutes

Yield: 20 – 24 servings

INGREDIENTS

- ½ cup peanut butter (almond butter works too)
- ⅓ Cup pure maple syrup*
- ¼ cup almond milk
- ¼ cup coconut oil
- tablespoons cacao, cocoa or Dutch cocoa
- 1 – 2 teaspoons vanilla

- 2 cups old fashioned oats (quick oats is fine too)

INSTRUCTIONS

1. Warm mixture: Start by warming the peanut butter, coconut oil, maple syrup, almond milk, vanilla and cacao powder over low heat, constantly stirring until warm and starting to thicken.

2. Remove from heat and stir in the oats and mix well to coat.

3. Drop 2 rounded tablespoonful of the mixture on a cookie sheet lined with parchment paper or Silpat. Shape them nicely and flatten the tops a little if you like, or simply leave them in rustic-looking mounds of chocolaty goodness.

4. Place the cookie sheet in the refrigerator to chill. You can grab one after 30 minutes, but they set up best after 6 hours in the fridge.

5. Recipe yields about 20 – 24 no bake cookies.

NOTES

Substitute maple syrup with coconut sugar or pure cane sugar. Just add 2 extra tablespoons of almond milk.

NUTRITION FACTS:

Calories: 24kcal | Carbohydrates: 15g | Protein: 22g | Fat: 9g | Saturated
Fat: 1g | Sodium: 69mg | Potassium: 446mg | Fiber: 6g | Sugar: 4g | Vitamin A: 1660IU | Vitamin C: 80mg | Calcium: 25mg | Iron: 3mg

BANANA CHIA PUDDING

Banana chia seed pudding in the cup with banana slices, coconut flakes and shaved chocolate. Easy banana chia seed pudding, with only 3 simple ingredients, is great for breakfast, dessert, or light snack!

Prep Time: 6 hours

Total Time: 6 hours

Yield: Serves 6

INGREDIENTS

- 2 large overripe bananas
- 2 cups unsweetened coconut (beverage), almond or cashew milk
- 6 tablespoons chia seeds
- Optional add-ins
- 2 – 4 tablespoons pure maple syrup
- ½ – 1 teaspoon vanilla extract
- To garnish
- Toasted coconut flakes
- Banana slices
- Cacao nibs or shaved dark chocolate

INSTRUCTIONS

1. In a medium bowl, add bananas and mash well, stir in non-dairy milk and chia seeds, mix well.
2. Let sit for about 30 minutes, and give a good stir, repeat one more time, stirring again after 30 minutes.

This step is important, as the seeds need to be stirred once or twice before completely gelling up and setting. If not stirred, the mixture will be soupy—cover and place in the refrigerator for at least 6 hours, or overnight.

3. Serve with sliced bananas, toasted coconut flakes and cacao nibs/shaved chocolate. Would also be great with a dollop of coconut whipped cream! Makes about 3 cups.

NOTES

Make this raw by using homemade nut milk of choice.

NUTRITION FACTS:

Calories: 224kcal | Carbohydrates: 15g | Protein: 32g | Fat: 9 g | Saturated Fat: 1g Sodium: 61mg Potassium: 46mg Fiber: 6g | Sugar: 4g | Vitamin A: 1660IU | Vitamin C: 80mg | Calcium: 255mg | Iron: 3mg

NO-BAKE RASPBERRY VEGAN CHEESECAKE

Simple, summery and brimming with raspberries inside and out! It's my kind of wonderful with this easy no bake vegan cheesecake.

Prep Time: 6 hours 15 min

Total Time: 6 hours 15 minutes

Yield: Serves 8 - 12

Category: Dessert, No Bake

INGREDIENTS

Crust

- 1 cup almonds, raw or toasted (old fashioned oats would be ok too)
- 1 cup Medjool dates (about 10), pitted and chopped
- Pinch of mineral salt

Filling

- cups raw cashews, soaked for 2 – 3 hours and drained
- ⅓ cup unsweetened vanilla cashew milk
- ⅓ – ½ cup pure maple syrup
- 1 heaping teaspoon vanilla powder or 1 teaspoon vanilla extract
- Pinch mineral salt
- 2 cups frozen or fresh raspberries

Toppings, optional

- Shaved dark chocolate or cacao nibs
- 1 – 2 cups frozen or fresh raspberries

INSTRUCTIONS

1. Crust: Place almonds, dates and salt in a food processor/blender, and blend until coarse. Line a round 8 × 8 or 9 × 9 pan or spring-foam pan with parchment paper or cling wrap. Add the nut crust to the pan and gently press against the bottom and around the corners, filling in as evenly as possible.

2. Rinse the food processor/blender and begin the filling.

3. Filling: Place the drained cashews, milk, maple syrup, vanilla and salt back in the food processor/blender, blend until smooth scraping down the sides as needed. Be patient and let the machine run a few minutes extra to be sure it's smooth. Add the raspberries to the filling and fold in by hand using a spatula. Add the mixture to the prepared pan, making sure to spread evenly filling in the entire pan. Gently tap pan on a flat, hard surface to remove air bubbles. Top with optional toppings (you can also add toppings after it's been frozen).

4. Freeze: Place in freezer for at least 6 hours to overnight.

5. Serve: Before serving, pull the cake from the pan and remove the parchment paper/cling wrap. Let set 5 – 10 minutes before slicing. Enjoy this easy, vegan cheesecake!

NOTES: If you'd like to cut down on the nuts, try using old-fashioned oats in place of the almonds when making the crust. Vary up the crust by adding 2 tablespoons of cacao powder for a chocolate version. Alternately, add in ¼ cup shredded coconut for a coconut flavor. And, if you feel like making it supreme, add both the cacao and coconut when making the crust for maximum flavor!

Make this raw by using homemade nut-milk.

NUTRITION FACTS:

Calories: 224kcal | Carbohydrates: 15g | Protein: 12g | Fat: 9 g | Saturated   Fat: 1g | Sodium: 39mg | Potassium: 56mg Fiber: 6g | Sugar: 4g Vitamin A: 1660IU Vitamin C: 60mg Calcium: 255mg Iron: 3mg

PEANUT BUTTER + CACAO NIBS RICE CRISPY TREATS

A fun, healthy snack anytime of the day that's super easy to put together and ready to eat in minutes. Gluten-free, oil-free, dairy-free and marshmallow free.

Prep Time: 5 min

Cook Time: 35 min

Total Time: 40 minutes

Yield: Makes 9 bars

INGREDIENTS

- 1 cup brown rice syrup
- 1 cup natural peanut butter
- 5 cups rice crispy cereal (I used One Degree)
- ⅓ Cup cacao nibs

INSTRUCTIONS

1. Line a 9 x 9 square pan (or 9 x 13 rectangular dish) with parchment paper. Alternately, lightly grease with coconut oil or non-dairy butter. Set aside.

2. In a large pot or pan, over low heat, gently warm the brown rice syrup and peanut butter, stirring frequently. Remove from heat, stir in the crispy rice cereal, mix until almost combined. Add in the cacao nibs, and continue mixing until well combined.

3. Place the mixture in the prepared pan/dish, and gently, but firmly, press until compacted and evenly distributed.

4. Both cut into squares and serve as is, or place pan/dish in the refrigerator for about 30 minutes to let harden.

5. Using a 9 x 9 dish will yield 9 bars.

NOTES: If you can't source One Degree Sprouted Brown Rice Cereal, feel free to use the original Rice Krispy Cereal for a true 'crispy' bar. There are a few other brands that have rice crispy cereal, I just haven't tried them all but feel free to use any brand you know and like.

Use creamy or chunky peanut butter. Sun butter would be great too.

NUTRITION FACTS:

Calories: 224kcal | Carbohydrates: 45g | Protein: 22g | Fat: 9g |

SNACKS

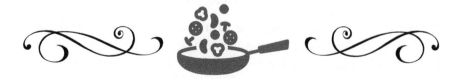

CHAI CHOCOLATE POPCORN (STOVETOP)

Chai Chocolate Popcorn made on the stovetop with hints of cocoa and warming chai spice, blended with a touch of sweetness makes for a delicious popcorn topping!

Prep Time: 5 min

Cook Time: 5 min

Total Time: 10 minutes

Yield: Makes 12, 1 cup servings

Category: Snack

INGREDIENTS

- tablespoons coconut oil
- ½ cup popcorn (pref. organic)
- 1 tablespoon sugar (coconut sugar or organic cane sugar)
- 1 tablespoon cocoa powder
- 1 ½ teaspoons cinnamon

- 1 teaspoon cardamom

- 1 teaspoon ground ginger

- ½ teaspoon clove or nutmeg

- Pinch of mineral salt + pepper, optional

INSTRUCTIONS

1. Spices: In a small bowl, mix your spices. Feel free to use heaping measurements.

2. Heat oil: In a large stockpot, add coconut oil, cover and heat over medium high heat for about 2 ½ minutes. Add popcorn: Pour popcorn into a pot and cover with lid, let cook for 2 – 3 minutes, carefully shaking the pot back and forth almost continuously. Popcorn will be done when you don't hear kernels popping for 5 – 10 seconds.

3. Add spice: Once popping comes to a minimum, lift the lid, add spices, cover tightly, carefully lift pot and tilt, round and round, upside down, every which way you can.

4. Serve: Enjoy right from the pot or pour popcorn in a large bowl or small individual bowls.

5. Makes about 12 to 14 cups

NOTES: - If you don't have all the spices, you can still make a flavorful topping using just a few...try simply using sugar, cocoa and cinnamon.

If you happen to have the Tazo Chai Teabags on hand, they will work too. Cut open 3 tea bags, combine with sugar and cocoa. Add once the popcorn is ready.

Feel free to omit the sugar or lessen it. If you omit the sugar, you may opt to add ¼ – ½ teaspoon black pepper for a more authentic chai spice.

Popcorn maker: Add popcorn, cook as directed and move to a large bowl. In a small bowl, melt coconut oil. Once the popcorn is done, drizzle with oil and top with seasoning, toss to coat well.

NUTRITION FACTS

Calories: 224kcal | Carbohydrates: 15g | Protein: 22g | Fat: 9g | Saturated
Fat: 1g | Sodium: 69mg | Potassium: 446mg | Fiber: 6g | Sugar : 4g | Vitamin A: 1660IU | Vitamin C: 80mg

STUFFED AVOCADOS

Both festive and fun, they make for a great snack, side or light meal. Enjoy the various ways to stuff your avocados!

Prep Time: 15 min

Total Time: 15 min

Yield: Serves 3 - 6 1x

Category: Side, Appetizer, Snack

INGREDIENTS

- avocados, sliced in half and seed removed

- 1 lemon, juice of

- ⅓ Cucumber, diced

- 1 bell pepper (any color), cored and diced

- 1 jalapeno, seeds removed and diced

- ¼ red onion or 1 small shallot, diced

- 1 garlic clove, minced or ⅛ – ¼ teaspoon garlic powder (optional)

- Small handful grape tomatoes, diced (optional)
- 2 – 4 tablespoons hummus, vegan mayo or garlic aioli
- Mineral salt & cracked pepper, to taste

INSTRUCTIONS

1. Prepare the ingredients. Once you've sliced the avocados and removed the seeds, squeeze or rub a little lemon juice on the flesh to keep the browning at bay.
2. Place the cucumber, bell pepper, jalapeno, onion, and optional garlic and diced tomatoes in a small/medium mixing bowl; add just enough of the hummus or vegan mayo to bind.
3. Fill avocados and top with salt, pepper and squeeze of lemon. Adding a little chopped parsley will add even more color!

NOTES: -To make raw, use this Raw Spouted Hummus.

Try adding in some freshly chopped herbs to your mixture. You may consider a little dill, oregano, basil, cilantro, etc.

NUTRITION FACTS:

Calories: 196 cal, Fat: 10g, Protein: 13g, Carbohydrate: 14g, Sugar: 6g, Fiber: 3g, Sodium: 567mg

FRESH CORN SALSA

Fresh Corn Salsa recipe is colorful, delicious and super easy to make. It's a perfect summer salsa and nice change up from tomato based salsa recipes.

Prep Time: 10 min Total Time: 10 min

Yield: Serves 8

INGREDIENTS

- ears of corn (about 3 ½ – 4 cups), shucked and cut from the cob
- 1 red bell pepper, cored and finely diced
- ½ red onion, finely diced
- 1 jalapeno, finely diced (a few seeds are ok for extra heat)
- 2 limes, juice of
- ¼ – ½ teaspoon chili powder, optional
- Generous pinch of mineral salt

INSTRUCTIONS

- Assemble: In a large mixing bowl, combine the corn, bell pepper, onion, jalapeno, lime juice and salt, mix well to combine. Taste for flavor adding more lime juice or salt to taste.
- Makes about 4 – 5 cups.

NOTES

Optional add-ins:

- For added creaminess add 1 avocado, diced
- For extra protein add 1 can (14oz) black beans (about 1 ½ cups), drained and rinsed
- Generous dash of cumin
- In place of jalapeno, try using hatch, poblano or Anaheim chili. Or for extra spicy, use serrano peppers.

- If fresh corn is unavailable, use frozen corn that has been thawed or canned corn (about 2 – 14oz. cans), drained of the juices.

- If you don't care for raw onions, 'deflame' them by cutting the onion into thin slices and soaking in hot water for 10 minutes before dicing.

NUTRITION FACTS:

Calories: 166 cal, Fat: 10g, Protein: 13g, Carbohydrate: 14g, Sugar: 6g, Fiber: 3g, Sodium: 507mg

LENTIL & SUN-DRIED TOMATO HUMMUS WRAP

Lentil Hummus Wrap with sun-dried tomato hummus, leafy greens and protein rich lentils is full of flavor and makes a great addition to the brown bag lunch!

Prep Time: 15 min Total Time: 15 min

Yield: Serves 3

INGREDIENTS

- Lavash bread (whole grain pref.) or flour tortillas

- ½ cup cooked lentils, per wrap

- Leafy greens (I used romaine)

- Red pepper flakes

- Mineral salt

- Sun-Dried Tomato Hummus

- 1 ½ cups fresh cooked garbanzo beans (chickpeas) or 1 can (15oz) garbanzo beans

- 2 – 3 tablespoons sun-dried tomatoes, chopped

- ¼ cup tahini (or cut in half and use 2 Tbsp extra virgin olive oil)

- 1 clove garlic

- ½ teaspoon paprika (regular or smoked)

- ½ teaspoon mineral salt, or to taste

- Juice of 1 lemon or 1 – 2 tablespoons lemon juice

- ¼ – ⅓ cup water, as needed

INSTRUCTIONS

Sun-Dried Tomato Hummus:

1. If using packaged sun-dried tomatoes, soak your tomatoes in water for about 15 minutes to soften, reserve water. If they are super fresh, no need to soak, just chop and use. Use the remaining water as needed when adding it to the hummus. If using bottled in oil sun-dried tomatoes, use as is.

2. Place all ingredients into the food processor/blender, except for the water. Blend until creamy, about 3 minutes or so, adding water as needed to thin. I used about ⅓ cup water as I like my hummus on the moist, thin side.

3. Makes about 1 ½ cups.

Assemble your wrap:

Lay your lavash bread on a flat surface. Spread a nice layer of hummus over ¾, top with about ½ cup lentils over the top, sprinkle with red pepper flakes and a mineral salt, add leafy greens over the top. Roll gently, but tightly as you can. Slice in half and enjoy!

NOTES

Feel free to play around with the tahini and olive oil adjusting to suit your taste. You may like more tahini, or you may not have any on hand and can use olive oil in its place.

If you're looking to make this virtually fat free, use water in place of the tahini and olive oil.

Store hummus tightly covered in the refrigerator for up to six days. Makes about 1 ½ cups.

Try this hummus with warmed corn tortillas or fresh sliced cucumbers, zucchini, carrots, bell peppers, etc. Thin a little more and use as a crema for tacos, enchiladas, and burritos. You can even use it in your salads! Hummus is so versatile and my new nut based cream replacements whenever possible!

NUTRITION FACTS:

Calories: 196 cal, Fat: 10g, Protein: 13g, Carbohydrate: 14g, Sugar: 6g

VEGAN COCONUT MACAROONS

Toasty coconut on the outside and tender on the inside, these vegan coconut macaroons use minimal ingredients and are super easy to make!

Prep Time: 15 min Cook Time: 25 min Total Time: 40 minutes

Yield: Makes 24

INGREDIENTS

- cups unsweetened coconut flakes, finely shredded (see notes)

- 1 cup canned coconut milk or cream, full or low-fat

- ⅓ cup pure maple syrup

- ⅓ cup slivered almonds (chopped is ok too), optional

- ⅓ cup oat flour, all-purpose, or gluten-free flour blend*

- 2 teaspoons vanilla extract

- Pinch of mineral salt

- 7 oz. vegan dark chocolate bar or chocolate chips

INSTRUCTIONS

1. Preheat oven to 350 degrees F. Line a baking sheet with parchment paper or a Silpat.

2. Mix: In a medium size mixing bowl, combine the coconut, coconut milk, syrup, almonds, flour, vanilla, and salt, mix well.

3. Scoop: Using a 2 or 3 tablespoons measuring spoon, scoop out rounded tablespoons, making sure to pack it well.

4. This last part is very important, or your macaroons may tend to fall apart. Place packed mounds on a cookie sheet, about 1 inch apart.

5. Bake: Place cookie sheet in the oven and bake for 20 – 30 minutes (ovens vary and it depends on how big the mounds are), until golden, rotating sheet halfway through baking. Let cool completely.

6. Chocolate: Warm the chocolate on the stove over low heat, frequently stirring until melted. Alternately, you can melt the chocolate in the microwave, stopping to give a good stir every 30 seconds. Dip the bottoms of the macaroons into the melted chocolate. Place the cookies back on the lined baking sheet. Drizzle

remaining chocolate on top using a spoon or pastry piping bag. Refrigerate for 7 – 10 minutes, or until set. Makes about 24 two tablespoon cookies, 18 three tablespoon cookies, or 12 four tablespoon coconut macaroons.

NOTES: Spelt, all-purpose and pastry flour is ok too. If using coconut flour, use ⅓ cup. **It** is very important to gently, but firmly, pack the mixture when making the coconut mounds. If they aren't packed well, they will likely fall apart or 'go flat' when done.

Use the right shredded coconut. There are different sizes of shredded coconut (large, medium and finely shredded). Make sure to use finely shredded (almost minced) for the same results here.

Maple syrup substitute: Use ½ cup of sugar and add an extra ¼ cup of coconut milk.

NUTRITION FACTS:

Calories: 196 cal, Fat: 10g, Protein: 10g, Carbohydrate: 14g, Sugar: 8g

BANANA CARAMEL BREAD PUDDING

Servings: 4

Prep Time: 10 mins Cooking Time: 30 mins

INGREDIENTS

- 2 large bananas, ripe
- 1/2 cup date paste
- 3/4 cup almond milk
- 2 teaspoons cinnamon

- 8 slices whole grain cinnamon raisin bread, cubed
- 1/2 cup coconut milk

DIRECTIONS

1. preheat oven to 375°F.
2. In a food processor or blender, add the bananas, date paste, almond milk, and cinnamon and blend until smooth.
3. Transfer to a large mixing bowl. Add the bread cubes to the mixing bowl and mix until well combined.
4. Divide the bread mixture into 4 ramekins, pour 2 tablespoons of coconut milk over each. Place in oven and bake for 30 minutes, or until bread is golden and caramelized.

NUTRITION FACTS:

- (Per Serving) Calories: 407
- Protein: 9 grams
- Carbohydrates: 83 grams
- Fat: 10 grams

ROASTED PINEAPPLE

Servings: 2 (3 slices per serving)

Prep Time: Under 5 mins

Cooking Time: 20 – 25 mins

INGREDIENTS

- 6 slices pineapple, about 1/2-inch thick

- 2 tablespoons brown sugar

DIRECTIONS

1. Preheat broiler. Coat a baking sheet in cooking spray.

2. Spread out the pineapple on the baking sheet and sprinkle with brown sugar. Broil for 10 – 15 minutes, or until golden brown. Flip and broil for another 5 – 10 minutes, until golden brown.

NUTRITION FACTS

- (Per Serving) Calories: 117

- Protein: 1 gram

- Carbohydrates: 31 grams

- Fat: 0 grams

CHOCOLATE SWEET POTATO PUDDING

Servings: 2

Prep Time: Under 5 mins

INGREDIENTS

- 1/2 medium sweet potato, cooked

- 1 medium avocado

- 5 dates, pitted and soaked

- 2 tablespoons carob or chocolate powder

- 1/4 cup water

DIRECTIONS

1. In a food processor or blender add all of the ingredients and pulse until ingredients are mostly mixed. Turn on high and slowly add any additional water until the pudding is smooth.

CRAN-STRAWBERRY POPSICLES

Servings: 8 Prep Time: 5 minutes

Chilling Time: 1 hour, or until set

INGREDIENTS

- 2 cups fresh strawberries
- 1/4 cup frozen cranberry juice concentrate, thawed
- 1 teaspoon stevia or another natural sweetener
- 1 tablespoon lemon juice
- tablespoons water

DIRECTIONS

1. In a blender or food processor, add the strawberries, cranberry concentrate, stevia, lemon juice, and water and process until smooth.

2. Pour the mixture into 8 Popsicle molds or small paper cups. Place in freezer until they begin to set, about 1 hour.

2. Insert Popsicle sticks and place back in the freezer until completely set.

NUTRITION FACTS

(Per Serving)

- Calories: 31
- Protein: 0 grams
- Carbohydrates: 8 grams
- Fat: 0 grams

REFRIED BEAN & AVOCADO LAVASH WRAP

A simple, vegan lavash wrap with refried beans, avocado, red bell pepper, onion, and salsa side is perfect for a healthy lunch, dinner or make ahead meal.

Prep Time: 5 min Cook Time: 5 min Total Time: 10 minutes

Yield: Serves 2

INGREDIENTS

- 2 Lavash bread (whole grain)
- 1 can (14 oz.) vegan refried beans
- ⅓ Red onion, sliced
- 1 large red bell pepper, sliced
- 1 head romaine lettuce or other leafy greens of choice
- ½ avocado, sliced
- Cilantro sprigs, optional
- Himalayan salt & pepper
- Salsa on the side

INSTRUCTIONS

3. Heat up your refried beans and cut up your veggies.

4. Layer lavash bread with ⅓ – ½ of the refried beans, onion, red pepper, avocado and leafy greens. Sprinkle a little mineral salt over the top, fold over and roll, slice in half and enjoy! A little salsa on the side is perfect for adding a little extra juiciness. You could also use tomato slices in place of, or in addition to, the red bell pepper for added juiciness.

NOTES

Use homemade refried beans made from scratch for the best flavor. Preferably, Instant Pot Refried Beans or Slow Cooker Refried Beans.

NUTRITION FACTS:

Calories: 156 cal, Fat: 10g, Protein: 13g, Carbohydrate: 14g, Sugar: 6g, Sodium: 56mg

PUMPKIN GRANOLA (VEGAN + OIL FREE)

Full of flavor and perfect for snacking, this crunchy pumpkin granola is naturally sweetened and made with only a handful of ingredients! It's oil-free, refined sugar-free and easy to make.

Prep Time: 5 min Cook Time: 30 min Total Time: 35 minutes

Yield: Serves 16

Category: Snack

Method: Oven, Bake

INGREDIENTS

- cups old fashioned oats

- 1 cup pecans

- ½ cup Pepitas

- 1 teaspoon cinnamon or pumpkin pie spice

- ¼ teaspoon allspice or nutmeg

- ¼ – ½ teaspoon mineral salt

- ⅔ Cup pure maple syrup

- ½ cup 100% pumpkin puree

- 1 teaspoon vanilla extract, optional

INSTRUCTIONS

- Prep: Preheat the oven to 300 degrees F. Line a baking sheet with parchment paper or a silicone mat.

- Dry ingredients: In a medium mixing bowl, combine the oats, pecans, pepitas and spices.

- Wet ingredients: In a measuring cup or small bowl, mix the pumpkin puree and maple syrup.

- Mix wet & dry: Pour the wet mixture into the dry ingredients, mix well to combine.

- Layer: Spread the granola on a rimmed baking sheet in a single layer.

- Bake: Place in the oven at bake for 40 – 50 minutes, stirring halfway through. Let cool; granola will harden as it cools.

- Makes about 4 ½ – 5 cups. Serves 16, about ⅓ cup per serving.

NOTES:

Additional add-ins:

- 1 – 2 teaspoon vanilla extract (mix in with wet ingredients)
- ½ cup coconut flakes (add to dry ingredients)

FUELING HACKS

GREEK YOGURT COOKIE DOUGH

INGREDIENTS

- Time: - 5 minutes
- I packet Optavia Essential Chewy Chocolate Chip Cookie
- 1.53.2 Oz container low fat plain Greek yogurt
- 1 serving
- 1 Fueling no leaner
- Combine all the ingredients (I packet Optavia Essential Chewy Chocolate Chip Cookie
- 1.53.2 Oz container low fat plain Greek yogurt) and chill until ready to serve.

NUTRITION FACTS

- Calories 248.0
- Total Carbohydrate 18.7 g

- Dietary Fiber 1.0 g

- Sugars15.6 g

- Protein   18.5 g

ZESTY TORTILLA CHIPS WITH GUACAMOLE

INGREDIENTS

Yield: - 2 servings

- Per Serving: - 1 fuelling 1 healthy fat 1 condiment

- Total time: - 30 minutes

- 2 sachets Optavia Hearty red bean and vegetable chili

- ¼ cup water

- Cooking Spray

GUACAMOLE

- oz peeled, pitted and mashed avocado

- I tbsp pico de gallo

- ½ tbsp of lime or lemon juice

- ⅛ tsp salt

INSTRUCTIONS

1. Preheat oven to 350F

2. Empty content of Hearty Red Bean and Veg Chili into a food processor and pulverize into a fine powder.

3. Transfer flour into a mixing bowl, add water and whisk until smooth

4. Place dough onto a piece of lightly greased parchment paper and use fingers to press into a ¼ inch thick circle. Use a pizza cutter to cut shaped tortilla pieces

5. Place the parchment paper with chips on a baking sheet. Bake for 10 minutes, flip and bake for another 10 to 15 minutes or until chips are crispy.

6. Meanwhile prepare the guacamole. Place mashed avocado in a small mixing bowl, and stir in the remaining ingredients. Refrigerate until ready to serve.

NUTRITION FACTS

- Total Fat 7ggrams 3%Saturated Fat 0.5ggrams

- Trans Fat 0ggrams 0%Cholesterol 0mgmilligrams 6%Sodium 140mgmilligrams

- 5%Total Carbohydrates 16ggrams 4%Dietary Fiber 1ggrams Sugars 1ggrams

- 0%Includes 0ggrams Added Sugars Protein 2g

HAMBURGER MAC

1 fueling, ½ lean/ 3 condiments.

1 serving

10 minutes

INGREDIENTS

- 1 sachet Optavia Cheesy Buttermilk mac

- I/2 tbsp tomato paste

- ¼ chili powder
- "" garlic powder
- "" onion powder
- 3oz cooked lean ground beef

INSTRUCTIONS

1. Prepare Optavia Cheesy Buttermilk mac according to package direction
2. While mac is still hot, stir in tomato sauce until smooth. Stir in beef and seasonings.

NUTRITION FACTS

- Cholesterol 0mg   0% Sodium 630mg 27%
- Total Carbohydrate 25g   9% Dietary Fiber < 1g 3%

CHIPOTLE MAC AND CHEESE WAFFLES

- 2 sachets Optavia select chipotle Mac and Cheese
- oz Coldwater
- 6 teaspoons liquid egg whites
- Cooking Spray
- 1 tbsp hot sauce
- 2 tbsp sugar free maple syrup (optional)

INSTRUCTIONS

1. In a medium-sized microwave safe bowl, mix Chipotle Mac and cheese and water until well combined. Microwave on high for 1&½ minutes, stir and let it stand for 1 minute, stir and let cool until cooled.whisk in liquid egg whites.

2. Pour mixture into hot, lightly greased waffle iron. Close the lid and bake for 3 to 5 minutes until cooked throughout. Carefully remove waffle from waffle iron and serve with hot sauce or maple syrup as desired.

NUTRITION FACTS:

- Cholesterol 0mg   0% Sodium 430mg 27%

CHOCOLATE PEANUT BUTTER DONUTS

Yield: 4 servings

Per Serving:- 1 fueling 1 condiment 1 and 1/4 OPTIONAL SNACK.

Time range: 20 minutes

INGREDIENTS

- 2 Optavia Golden Essential Golden dip chocolate pancakes

- 2 Optavia Golden Essential Decadent Double Chocolate Brownie

- 6 tsp liquid eggs substitute

- ¼ cup unsweetened vanilla almond or cashew milk

- ½ tsp vanilla extract

- ½ tsp baking powder
- Cooking Spray.
- For glaze
- ¼ powdered peanut butter
- 3-4 unsweetened vanilla almond or cashew milk

INSTRUCTIONS

1. Preheat oven to 350F

2. Sift out chocolate chip pancakes and set aside (optional). In a medium sized bowl, combine pancakes, egg substitute, vanilla extract, milk, and baking powder. Divide mixture evenly amongst four slots of a donut pan, and bake until mixture is set about 10-15 minutes. Let cool before glazing.

3. Meanwhile prepare peanut butter glaze in a small shallow bowl. Combine powdered peanut butter and milk until smooth and slightly runny. Dip each baked pancake into the glaze and top chocolate chips.

NUTRITION FACTS

Calories 34. Total Fat 0.62. Cholesterol 2.15. Sodium 41.25. Potassium 24.14.

Total Carbohydrate 4.58. Protein 2.43.

SWEET POTATO MECCAN MUFFINS

Yield: 4 servings

Per Serving:- 1 healthy fat, 1 condiment and 1 fueling

Total time: 30 minutes

INGREDIENTS

- 2 sachets Optavia select honey sweet potatoes
- 1 cup cold water
- 2 sachets Optavial Spiced Gingerbread
- 6 tbsp liquid egg substitute
- ¼ unsweetened vanilla almond or cashew milk
- ½ tbsp pumpkin pie spice
- ½ tsp vanilla extract
- ½ tsp baking powder
- Cooking Spray
- Chopped Pecans

INSTRUCTIONS

1. Pre-heat oven to 350F
2. Prepare Honey Sweet Potatoes according to package directions. Let cool slightly
3. In a medium sized bowl, combine cooked honey sweet potatoes and remaining ingredients (except for the pecans)...
4. Divide mixture amongst eight slots of lightly greased standard sized muffin pans. Sprinkle top with chopped pecans—Bake for 30 minutes.

NUTRITION FACTS

Cholesterol 1.5mg - Sodium 51.1mg 3% Potassium 233.4mg -

Carbohydrates 13.2g   - Net carbs 11.6g   - Sugar 3.6g
    - Fiber 1.6g   7%

Glucose 0.2g Fructose 0.2g Lactose 0g Maltose 0.9g Galactose 0g Sucrose 2.1g Protein 14g

OATMEAL BARS

INGREDIENTS

- 1 Fueling and 1 Condiment
- 1 Octavia Oatmeal Packet (1 Fueling)
- 1 tbsp egg beaters
- 2 tbsp vanilla sugar free syrup (1 Condiment)
- tbsp water

INSTRUCTIONS

1. Preheat oven to 350 degrees. Stir ingredients together. Let sit for 5 minutes. Pour into a ramekin. Bake for 12 minutes or microwave for 1 minute in a 1200 watt microwave. Cool. Cut into bars.

2. 1 Fueling and 1 Condiment

PUDDING PIES

- 2 Servings with 1 Meal and 1 Condiment per Serving
- Ingredients:
- 1 Packet of Octavia Maple and Brown Sugar Oatmeal (any flavor can be used)
- 1 Packet of Octavia Banana Pudding (any flavor can be used)

- 1 Packet of Splenda (1 condiment)

- 1/2 tsp Baking Powder (1 condiment)

INSTRUCTIONS

1. Preheat oven to 350 degrees.

2. Mix oatmeal, Splenda and baking powder. Slowly add water until the dough just sticks together. I used about 1/2 cup of water, but it can vary. Divide the dough into 2 balls and press into two ramekins sprayed with Pam. Bake at 350 degrees for 12 minutes. Let completely cool. Using the shaker jar, mix 4 oz of water with the banana pudding. Spoon into each oatmeal cup. Refrigerate for about 30 minutes for it to set.

CINNAMON ROLL WITH CREAM CHEESE ICING

INGREDIENTS

- 1 pancake mix (1 Fueling)

- 2 tbsp water

- 1/8 tsp cinnamon (1/4 Condiment)

- 1 tbsp light cream cheese (1 Condiment)

- 1 packet Stevia, divided (1 Condiment)

- Cooking Spray Not Butter Spray (if you have a healthy fat to use up, you can have 10 sprays as 1 Healthy Fat)

INSTRUCTIONS

1. Combine pancake mix, cinnamon, half packet of Stevia, and water. Pour into a small container. Microwave for 50 seconds. Make sure you do not overcook it otherwise it will get dry. Spray the pancake with ICBINB spray. In the same bowl you used to make the pancake batter, combine cream cheese and the rest of the Splenda. Mix around with the little bit of batter that was left in the bowl. This adds a bit of the cinnamon mixture to the cream cheese. Spread on the pancake.

2. 1 Fueling, 2.25 Condiments and 1 Healthy Fat if you used the Butter Spray

NUTRITION FACTS:

1. Total calories: 133
2. Protein: 5
3. Carbs: 28
4. Fiber: 9.5
5. Fat: 1

ZUCCHINI BREAD

INGREDIENTS:

- Any Pancake packet (1 Fueling)
- 1/4 c. shredded zucchini (squeeze out the liquid by rolling in paper towels and squeezing) (1/2 of 1 Green)
- 2 tbsp egg beaters
- 1.5 oz water

- 1 packet Stevia (1 Condiment)

INGREDIENTS

Mix and bake in whatever style you'd like. I did it on the waffle iron, super-fast and yummy zucchini bread waffle. Consider mini muffins next, or even as just a pancake. If you decide to bake these, bake at 350 degrees. The time will vary depending on what type of pan you are using.

- 1 Serving with
- 1 Fueling, 1/2 of 1 Green, and 1 Condiment
- Cody Jo's Kinda Cadbury Creme Eggs
- **For Octavia Fudge:**
- 1 packet Octavia Hot Cocoa (1 Fueling)
- 2 TB Water
- **For Creme of Egg:**
- 1 TB Walden Farms Marshmallow Creme (1/2 Condiment)
- 1 tbsp PB2 (1/2 Snack)
- **For Outside of Egg**:
- 1 tbsp Walden Farms Chocolate Syrup - Optional (1/2 Condiment)

INSTRUCTIONS

1. Combine hot cocoa mix and 2 tbsp water until blended. Spoon half of the mixture on a plate and form an oval shape.

2. Combine ingredients PB2 and marshmallow creme. No need to add any water. You want the center to be a

little thick. Just make sure it is blended. Spoon on top of the half oval shape in the center. Top with the remaining half of the hot cocoa mixture, forming an oval egg shape. Spread 1 tbsp chocolate syrup over the top of the egg. Freeze for at least 20 minutes.

3. 1 Fueling, 1/2 Snack and 1 Condiment

You can use this guide to add up the ingredients you used:

- 1 TB Low Fat Cream Cheese = 1 Condiment

- 1 TB Full Fat Cream Cheese = 1 Healthy Fat

- 1 packet Stevia = 1 Condiment

- 1 TB Walden Farms Caramel or Chocolate Syrup = 1/2 Condiment

- 1 TB Marshmallow Creme = 1/2 Condiment

- 1 TB PB2 = 1/2 snack

MOUSSE TREAT

INGREDIENTS:

- 1 packet of MF hot cocoa (1 Fueling)

- 1/2 cup pre-made sugar free gelatin (cherry/strawberry) (1 Snack)

- 1 tbsp light cream cheese (1 Condiment)

- 2 tbsp to 1/4 cup cold water

- A little bit of crushed ice (about 1/4cup) - about 75% of it.

INSTRUCTIONS

- Mix it all in a bullet style blender.

- Has a nice rich creamy texture! ENJOY!

- 1 Fueling, 1 Optional Snack, and 1 Condiment

NUTRITION FACTS

- Total calories: 611 Protein: 13

- Carbs: 85

- Fiber: 5.25

- Fat: 1

TIRAMISU MILKSHAKE

Yield: 1 serving

INGREDIENTS

- 1fueling ½ leaner and 1&1/2 lean 2&½ condiment

- Total time: 5 minutes

- 1 sachet Optavia Frosty Coffee Soft serve treat

- ½ cup ice

- 6oz plain low fat Greek yogurt

- ½ cup of unsweetened vanilla almond or cashew milk

- 2 tbsp sugar free chocolate syrup

- 2tbsp pressurized whipped topping

INSTRUCTIONS

- Combine all ingredients in a blender and blend until smooth.

- Pour into a glass or Mason jar. Drizzle with syrup and top with whipped toppings.

NUTRITION FACTS:

Serving: 11/2 cups, Calories: 263kcal, Carbohydrates: 11g, Protein: 35g, Fat: 9g, Saturated Fat: 3g, Cholesterol: 96mg, Sodium: 485mg, Fiber: 4g, Sugar: 3.5g

GINGERBREAD TRIFLE

Yield: 4 servings

Per servings:- 1 fueling, ½ lean, 1&½ condiments

Total times:- 15 minutes

INGREDIENTS

- 2 sachets Optavial Essential Spibed Gingerbread

- 2 sachets "" "" Creamy Vanilla Shake

- 12oz plain low-fat Greek yoghurt

- ½ cup pressurized whipped topping such as Reddi whip

- ¼ cuo of sugar free salted caramel toffee or gingerbread syrup

INSTRUCTIONS

- Prepare Sliced Gingerbread according to package directions. Allow to cool and then cut into.small cubes

- In a mixing bowl, beat creamy vanilla shake wory Greek yoghurt

- Evenly divide the yoghurt mixture and cake cubes amongst four small trìfles or parfait dishes. Top with whipped topping and drizzle with syrup.

NUTRITION FACTS

Calories: 261kcal, Carbohydrates: 8g, Protein: 31g, Fat: 11.5g , Saturated Fat: 3.5g, Cholesterol: 83mg, Sodium: 658mg, Fiber: 3g, Sugar: 1g

TROPICAL SMOOTHIE BOWL

YIELD: - 1 serving

Per Serving: - 1 fueling 2 Healthy Fats 2 & ½ condiments

Total time: - 5 minutes

- 1 sachet Optavia Essential Tropical Fruit Smoothie

- ½ cup unsweetened, original coconut milk

- ½ cup ice

- ½ oz macadamias or cashews, chopped.

- 1 tbsp shredded, Unsweetèned coconut

- ½ tbsp Chia Seeds

- ½ tbsp lime zest

INSTRUCTIONS

1. Add Tropical Fruit Smoothie, milk and ice to a blender. Blend until smooth

2. Pour smoothie into a small, shallow bowl

3. Top with remaining ingredients, and serve.

NUTRITION FACTS:

Total calories: 103 Protein: 5 Carbs: 28 Fiber: 9.5 Fat: 0

YOGHURT BERRY BAGELS WITH CREAM CHEESE

Yield: - 2 servings

1 fueling, ½ healthy fat and 1 &½ condiments

Total time: 20 minutes

INGREDIENTS

- 2 sachets Essential Yogurt Berry Blast Smoothie
- ½ cup unsweetened original almond or cashew milk
- 2 tbsp liquid egg substitute
- ½ tsp baking powder
- Cooking Spray
- 1 oz light cream cheese

INSTRUCTIONS

1. Preheat oven to 350F
2. In a medium sized bowl, combine packets of yogurt Berry Blast Smoothie, egg substitute and baking powder.
3. Divide mixture among four, lightly greased slots of a donut pan
4. Bake until mixture is set, about 12 to 15 minutes.
5. Let cool slightly, before serving with cream cheese.

NUTRITION FACTS

Total calories: 611 Protein: 13 Carbs: 85 Fiber: 5.25 Fat: 1

KATIE'S PB BROWNIE ICE CREAM SANDWICHES

- Ingredients:
- 1 Brownie Mix (1 Fueling)
- 1 Peanut Butter Crunch Bar or any other bar you like such as Smores, Chocolate, etc. (1 Fueling)
- tbsp water
- 2 tbsp PB2 (1 Snack)
- 1 tbsp water
- 2 tbsp cool whip (2 Condiments)

INSTRUCTIONS

1. Melt 1 brownie and 1 peanut butter crunch for 20 seconds.
2. Add 3 tbsp water and mix. Spray a plate with cooking spray.
3. Drop 4 spoonfuls of dough on a plate.
4. Microwave for 2 minutes. Mix PB2 and water to form a paste.
5. Add peanut butter mixture to each of two cookies and then add 1 tbsp of cool whip to each of the other two cookies.
6. Place peanut butter cookie on top of the cookie with whip cream.

7. Place stuffed cookies in a Ziploc container and freeze thoroughly. Each cookie is one meal.

8. 2 Servings with 1 Fueling, 1 Condiment, and 1/2 Snack per serving

NUTRITION FACTS:

Total calories: 133 Protein: 5 Carbs: 28 Fiber: 9.5 Fat: 1

HONEY MUSTARD CHICKEN NUGGETS WITH MUSTARD DIPPING SAUCE

Yield:- 2 servings

Per Servings:- 1 lean/ 1 fueling/ 2 condiments

Total time:- 25 minutes

INGREDIENTS

- 12 oz boneless, skinless chicken breast, cubed
- 1 egg, beaten
- 2 sachets Optavia Essential Honey Mustard & Onion sticks, finely crushed to bread-crumb like consistency.
- ¼ cup plain low fat Greek yogurt
- 2 tsp spicy brown mustard
- ¼ tsp garlic powder
- Cooking Spray.

INSTRUCTIONS

1. Preheat oven to 400F

2. Place eggs and crushed Honey Mustard and Onion stick into two separate, small shallow bowls. Dip each chicken piece into the egg and then roll into the Crushed Honey Mustard and Onion Sticks until completely coated. Place chicken pieces onto a lightly greased foil-lined baking sheet. SPRAY top with cooking spray.

3. Bake until coating turns golden and internal temperature reaches 165F, about 18 to 20 minutes flipping halfway through.

4. Meanwhile, combine Greek yoghurt, mustard and garlic powder in a small bowl. Serve nuggets with yogurt dip.

NUTRITION FACTS:

Serving: 11/2

cups, Calories: 263kcal, Carbohydrates: 11g, Protein: 35g, Fat: 9g, Saturated

Fat: 3g, Cholesterol: 96mg, Sodium: 485mg, Fiber: 4g, Sugar

: 3.5g

PINA COLADA SHAKE

1 Fueling and 1/2 Condiment

INGREDIENTS:

- 1 MF Vanilla Shake (1 Fueling)

- 1/4 cup plus 2 tbsp water

- -4 ice cubes
- 1/2 cup diet ginger ale
- 1/4 tsp pineapple extract (1/4 Condiment)
- 1/8 tsp coconut extract (1/8 Condiment)
- 1/8 tsp rum extract (1/8 Condiment)

INSTRUCTIONS

Blend all ingredients together and serve.

FAUX-FRIED ZUCCHINI

INGREDIENTS

- 1 Medifast Cream of Broccoli Soup (1 Meal)
- 1½ cups zucchini, thinly sliced (3 greens)
- 2 teaspoons olive oil (2 healthy fats)
- ¼ teaspoon black pepper (1/2 condiment)
- ¼ teaspoon garlic powder (1 condiment)
- Non-stick cooking spray

INSTRUCTIONS

- Preheat oven to 400° F.
- Coat zucchini slices in olive oil.
- In a gallon Ziploc bag, combine the soup and spices.
- Toss zucchini slices in and shake to coat.
- Marinate in the refrigerator for 10 minutes.

- Coat a cookie sheet with non-stick cooking spray and lay out zucchini in a single layer.
- Bake for 12 minutes, or until brown along the edges.

NUTRITION FACTS:

Calories: 261kcal, Carbohydrates: 8g, Protein: 31g, Fat: 11.5g , Saturated Fat: 3.5g, Cholesterol: 83mg, Sodium: 658mg, Fiber: 3g, Sugar: 1g

SKINNY PEPPERMINT MOCHA

1 serving

I lean

1& ½ condiments

Time: - 5 minutes

INGREDIENTS

- One sachet Optavia Essential Velvety Hot Chocolate
- 6oz freshly brewed coffee
- ¼ cup of unsweetened vanilla almond or cashew milk (warmed)
- ¼ tsp peppermint extract
- 2 tbsp peppermint extract
- 2 tbsp pressurized whipped topping
- Pinch cinnamon

INSTRUCTIONS

1. Combine the first three INGREDIENTS in a mug or a coffee cup and stir until the velvety hot chocolate is dissolved.

2. Top with whipped topping and sprinkle with cinnamon

NUTRITION FACTS

Calories: 261kcal, Carbohydrates: 8g, Protein: 31g, Fat: 11.5g , Saturated Fat: 3.5g, Cholesterol: 83mg

CHICKEN NOODLE SOUP CHIPS

INGREDIENTS

- 1 packet Optavia Chicken Noodle Soup or any other soup or mac and cheese or chili will work (1 Fueling)

- Tbsp water

- Cooking spray

- Parchment paper

INSTRUCTIONS

1. Preheat oven to 375 degrees. Combine chicken noodle soup and any seasonings you want to use in a small blender. Pulse until it's a fine powder. In a small bowl, add the ground up soup and water, forming a small dough ball. Let sit for a few minutes.

2. Place the ball of dough on parchment paper that is lightly sprayed with cooking spray. Fold parchment over the dough and roll the dough as thin as possible or flatten it with your hands. The thinner it is, the

more crispy it gets. Carefully peel the parchment paper from the top of the dough and trim off any excess parchment paper. Place on a cookie sheet. Bake for about 10 minutes and remove from oven.

3. Using a sharp knife or your fingers, break into chips. Then spread the chips across the cookie sheet and bake for an additional 6 to 8 min or until crispy. Some chips may get done faster than others! That's okay! Just take the crispy ones out and finish baking the rest. They should be golden brown. Enjoy this tasty snack!

Makes **1 Serving**

Each serving provides **1 Fueling**

You can also microwave these chips by spreading the mixture thin on a flat plate—microwave 2 minutes. Flip and then microwave an additional *30 seconds* or until crispy.

NUTRITION FACTS

- Total Fat 2.8g 4 % Saturated Fat 0.9g   4   % Cholesterol 37mg   12 %

- Sodium 2204mg 96 % Total Carbohydrate 72g 26 % Dietary Fiber 3.7g   13 %

- Sugar 9.3g Protein 9.3g   19 %

GRILLED CHEESE TOMATO SANDWICH

INGREDIENTS

- 1 packet Octavia Cream of Tomato Soup (1 Fueling)

- 1/4 cup egg beaters (1/8 or .125 Lean)

- 1 slice 2% Reduced Fat American cheese (1/5 or .20 Lean)

INSTRUCTIONS

1. Mix soup and egg beaters together.

2. Pour evenly among the 4 squares of a sandwich maker—Cook for 3 minutes.

3. Fold in half and add cheese in the middle. Enjoy!

4. 1 Fueling and 1/3 Lean

NTRITION FACTS:

Cholesterol 37mg   12 %

Sodium 2204mg   96 % Total Carbohydrate 72g   26 %
Dietary Fiber 3.7g   13 %

Sugar 9.3g   Protein 9.3g 19 %

PIZZA BREAD

INGREDIENTS

- 1 Cream of Tomato Soup (1 Fueling)
- 1/4 tsp Baking Powder (1/2 Condiment)
- 2 tbsp Water
- 1/4 cup shredded reduced fat cheese (1/4 Lean)
- 1 Light Laughing Cow Cheese Wedge (1 Condiment)

INSTRUCTIONS

- Preheat oven to 425 degrees. Spray a cookie sheet with pam or use parchment paper. Combine soup, baking powder, seasonings and water. Spread the batter on a prepared cookie sheet and form a circle. I wet my hands and used them to spread the batter because the batter kept sticking to my spoon. Bake for 5 minutes and then flip using a spatula. If you would like to add cheese, do it now after flipping. Stick the bread back in the oven for 5 more minutes. If using laughing cow cheese, spread it on when the bread is done baking. Enjoy!

- 1 Fueling and 1/2 of a Condiment for Pizza Bread.

NUTRITION FACTS:

Serving: 11/2cups, Calories: 263kcal, Carbohydrates: 11g, Protein: 35g, Fat: 9g, Saturated
Fat: 3g, Cholesterol: 96mg, Sodium: 485mg, Fiber: 4g, Sugar: 3.5g

HAYSTACKS

INGREDIENTS:

- 1 Optavia Hot Cocoa or Brownie Mix (1 Fueling)
- 1 Optavia Cinnamon Pretzel Sticks, crushed (1 Fueling)
- tbsp water
- 2 tbsp PB2 (1 Optional Snack)
- 1 packet Stevia - optional (1 Condiment)

INSTRUCTIONS

- Crush the pretzels by opening one side of the bag and squeezing the bag to form crumbs. In a small bowl, combine hot cocoa or brownie mix with 3 tbsp of water to form a paste. Add 1 tbsp PB2 and Stevia; stir until combined. Add the crushed pretzels to the mixture and stir making sure the pretzels are evenly coated. Drop the haystacks on a piece of foil or plate forming 6 piles. Freeze for at least 30 minutes to an hour.

- 2 Servings with
- 1 Fueling, 1/2 Condiment and 1/2 Snack per Serving.

NUTRITION FACTS:

- Total Fat 8g - Saturated fat 2g - Cholesterol 20mg
- Sodium 1150mg 48% Carbohydrates 19g - Net carbs 17g - Sugar 2g - Fiber 2g   8%

GARLIC POTATO PANCAKES

INGREDIENTS:

- 1 Garlic Mashed Potatoes (1 Fueling)
- 1/4 tsp baking powder (1/2 Condiment)
- 1/4 cup reduced fat cheese, optional (1/4 Lean)
- 1/2 cup water

INSTRUCTIONS

1. Combine mashed potatoes, baking powder, water and cheese.
2. Let stand for 5 minutes so mixture can thicken up.
3. Lightly spray a cast iron skillet with cooking spray.
4. Heat skillet over medium heat.

5. Spoon mixture onto skillet forming two pancakes.

6. Cook for a few minutes and then flip the pancakes to cook the other side.

7. Serve with a tbsp of reduced sugar ketchup or 2 tbsp sour cream!

8. Makes 1 Serving

9. Each serving provides

10. 1 Fueling, 1/2 Condiment, and 1/4 Lean (if using cheese)

Additional Condiments:

- 1 tbsp Heinz Reduced Sugar Ketchup is 1 Condiment

- 1 tbsp sour cream ~ regular or light (1 Condiment)

- 2 tbsp sour cream is 1 Healthy Fat

NUTRITION FACTS:

Serving Size: 1/10 of the recipe

Calories: 262

Sugar: 29g

Sodium: 4mg

Fat: 7.5g

Saturated Fat: 0.7g

Carbohydrates: 46.8g

Fiber: 5.5g

Protein: 5.3g

PEANUT BUTTER BROWNIE WHOOPIE PIES

Yield:- 2 servings (2 whoopie pies per serving)

Per Servings:- 1 fuelling / ½ healthy fat/ 1 condiment/ 1 optional Snack

Total time: 25 minutes

INGREDIENTS

- 2 sachets Optavia Decadent Double Chocolate Brownie
- ¼ tsp of baking powder
- tbsp liquid egg substitute
- 6 tbsp unsweetened vanilla almond or cashew milk, divided
- 1tbsp veg Oil
- ¼ cup powdered peanut butter
- Cooking Spray

INSTRUCTIONS

1. Preheat oven to 350F

2. In a medium sized bowl, combine Decadent Double Chocolate Brownie mixture, baking powder, ¼ egg substitute, ¼ cup milk and oil and mix until a batter like consistency.

3. Divide batter evenly among four slots of a lightly greased muffin tin (should fill only a third of each slot). Bake until a toothpick inserted in centers comes out clean, about 18 to 20 minutes

4. Meanwhile, combine powdered peanut butter and remaining milk.

5. Once cooled, slice each muffin in half hour horizontally.

6. Spread one tbs poonpesnut butter filling unto the bottom half of each muffin and top with the remaining muffin halves. Enjoy!

MEAL PLANS

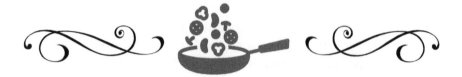

CLEAN EATING MEAL PLANS

14-Day Clean-Eating Meal Plan: 1,200 Calories

This easy clean-eating meal plan for weight loss features healthy whole foods and limits processed items to help you get back on track with healthy habits.

If you feel like your healthy habits have gotten off track, this simple take on a clean-eating meal plan can help you get back to the eating habits that help you feel your best. Throughout this 14-day diet plan, you'll get your fill of whole healthy foods-some that you will prepare from scratch and others that you can buy from the store at Octavia packages.

The meals and snacks in this plan will have you feeling energized, satisfied and good about what's on your plate. And at 1,200 calories, this diet meal plan will set you up to lose upwards of 4 pounds over the 2 weeks.

Need a higher calorie level? See this same clean-eating meal plan at 1,500 and 2,000 calories.

Clean-Eating Meal Plan for Beginners

If you're new to clean eating, the premise is simple—and following a meal plan (or simply using it for inspiration) can make it even easier to understand what it's all about. Clean-eating is a great way to up your intake of good-for-you foods (like whole grains, lean protein, healthy fats and plenty of fruits and veggies), while limiting the stuff that can make you feel not-so-great in large amounts (think refined carbs, alcohol, added sugars and hydrogenated fats).

While all foods can be part of a healthy diet, sometimes you just need to hit reset and focus on eating more of the healthy foods you may be skimping on. With 14 days of wholesome meals and snacks, this easy-to-follow clean-eating meal plan is a great way get more of those good for you foods.

If 14 days feel like too much, start with our 3-Day Clean Eating Kick-Start Meal Plan and go from there. Once you conquer this 14-day plan, try our Clean-Eating Challenge for 30 days, where you can plan to eat tons of delicious clean-eating foods, like what you will find in this meal plan.

Week 1

How to Meal Prep Your Week of Meals:

A little prep at the beginning of the week goes a long way to make the rest of the week easy.

DAY 1

Breakfast (287 calories)

> 1 serving Muesli with Raspberries

- Clean-Eating Shopping Tip: When buying muesli, look for a brand that doesn't have added sugars, which take away from the healthy goodness of this whole-grain breakfast.

- A.M. Snack (62 calories)

> 1 medium orange

- Lunch (360 calories)

  4 cups White Bean & Veggie Salad

- P.M. Snack (95 calories)

  1 medium apple

Dinner (420 calories)

- 4 cups (1 1/2 servings) Kale Salad with Beets & Wild Rice
- 1 serving Balsamic-Dijon Chicken

Daily Totals: 1,224 calories, 61 g protein, 153 g carbohydrates, 40 g fiber, 47 g fat, 1,400 mg sodium.

Day 2

Squash & Red Lentil Curry

Breakfast (270 calories)

- 1 serving Avocado-Egg Toast

  Clean-Eating Shopping Tip: Use sprouted-grain bread as your bread for these next two weeks as it's made without added sugars, unlike many store-bought pieces of bread. Also, if you plan to top your egg toast with hot sauce, look for a brand that's made without added sugars.

- A.M. Snack (101 calories)

  1 medium pear

- Lunch (392 calories)

  1 serving Greek Meatball Mezze Bowl

- P.M. Snack (62 calories)

  1 medium orange

- Dinner (439 calories)

  1 serving cup Squash & Red Lentil Curry

  1/2 cup Easy Brown Rice

Daily Totals: 1,225 calories, 63 g protein, 147 g carbohydrates, 33 g fiber, 46 g fat, 1,965 mg sodium.

Day 3

- Breakfast (287 calories)

  1 serving Muesli with Raspberries

- A.M. Snack (62 calories)

  1 medium orange

- Lunch (392 calories)

  1 serving Greek Meatball Mezze Bowl

- P.M. Snack (92 calories)

  12 almonds

- Dinner (439 calories)

  1 serving Asian Tilapia with Stir-Fried Green Beans

  1 cup Easy Brown Rice

Daily Totals: 1,206 calories, 62 g protein, 174 g carbohydrates, 37 g fiber, 48 g fat, 1,444 mg sodium.

Day 4

- Breakfast (257 calories)

  1/2 cup rolled oats, cooked in 1 cup milk

  1 medium plum, chopped

Cook oats and top with plum and a pinch of cinnamon.

- A.M. Snack (95 calories)

  1 medium apple

- Lunch (392 calories)

  1 serving Greek Meatball Mezze Bowl

- P.M. Snack (105 calories)

  1 medium banana

- Dinner (432 calories)

  1 serving Sheet-Pan Chicken & Brussels Sprouts

  1 1/2 cups mixed greens dressed with 2 Tbsp. Lemon-Tahini Dressing

Daily Totals: 1,214 calories, 58 g protein, 166 g carbohydrates, 32 g fiber, 41 g fat, 1,553 mg sodium.

Day 5

Greek Meatball Mezze Bowls

- Breakfast (290 calories)

  1 serving Peanut Butter-Banana Cinnamon Toast

  Clean-Eating Shopping Tip: When choosing store-bought peanut butter, avoid brands with added sugars and trans fats. Read more about choosing healthy peanut butter.

- A.M. Snack (32 calories)

  1/2 cup raspberries

- Lunch (392 calories)

  1 serving Greek Meatball Mezze Bowl

- Dinner (543 calories)

  1 serving Pork Chops with Garlicky Broccoli

Daily Totals: 1,225 calories, 54 g protein, 102 g carbohydrates, 30 g fiber, 71 g fat, 1,175 mg sodium.

Day 6

- Breakfast (257 calories)

  1/2 cup rolled oats, cooked in 1 cup milk

  1 medium plum, chopped

  Cook oats and top with plum and a pinch of cinnamon.

- A.M. Snack (101 calories)

  1 medium pear

- Lunch (325 calories)

  1 serving Veggie & Hummus Sandwich

- P.M. Snack (62 calories)

  1 medium orange

- Dinner (543 calories)

  1 serving Cauliflower rice-stuffed Peppers

  2 cups mixed greens dressed with 1 Tbsp. Citrus Vinaigrette

Daily Totals: 1,203 calories, 57g protein, 146 g carbohydrates, 31 g fiber, 49 g fat, 1,120 mg sodium.

Day 7

Mexican Cabbage Soup

- Breakfast (307 calories)

  2 cups Avocado Green Smoothie

- A.M. Snack (35 calories)

  1 Pancakes

- Lunch (352 calories)

  2 1/4 cup Tomato, Cucumber & White-Bean Salad with Basil Vinaigrette

  1 slice sprouted-grain bread, toasted and topped with 1 Tbsp. hummus

Meal-Prep Tip: Save a serving of the Tomato, Cucumber & White-Bean Salad with Basil Vinaigrette to have for lunch on Day 10. Store the dressing separately.

- P.M. Snack (30 calories)

  1 plum

- Dinner (490 calories)

  1 1/2 cups Mexican Cabbage Soup

  2 cups No-Cook Black Bean Salad

Daily Totals: 1,214 calories, 35 g protein, 163 g carbohydrates, 48 g fiber, 55 g fat, 1,365 mg sodium.

Week 2 weight loss

How to Meal Prep Your Week of Meals:

A little prep at the beginning of the week goes a long way to make the rest of your week easy.

Make a batch of the Meal-Prep Sheet-Pan Chicken Thighs and Basic Quinoa when preparing the Greek Kale Salad with Quinoa & Chicken recipe for dinner on Day 8. This way, you'll have leftover chicken and quinoa to use during the week. Store leftovers of the chicken and quinoa separately in large glass meal-prep containers.

Day 8

- Breakfast (338 calories)

  1 serving Scrambled Eggs with Vegetables
- A.M. Snack (119 calories)

  1/4 cup hummus

  1 cup sliced cucumber
- Lunch (325 calories)

  1 serving Veggie & Hummus Sandwich
- P.M. Snack (30 calories)

  1 plum
- Dinner (302 calories)

  1 serving Greek Kale Salad with Quinoa & Chicken
- Evening Snack (102 calories)

  1 serving Broiled Mango

Daily Totals: 1,216 calories, 58 g protein, 121 g carbohydrates, 26 g fiber, 60 g fat, 1,816 mg sodium.

Day 9

- Breakfast (307 calories)

  2 cups Jason Avocado Green Smoothie

  A.M. Snack (35 calories)

  1 pancake
- Lunch (328 calories)

1 1/2 cups Mexican Cabbage Soup

1 cup No-Cook Black Bean Salad

- P.M. Snack (92 calories)

  3/4 cup Kiwi & Mango with Fresh Lime Zest

- Dinner (453 calories)

  1 cup riced cauliflower, heated

  1 serving Soy-Lime Roasted Tofu

  2 cups Colorful Roasted Sheet-Pan Veggies

  1 Tbsp. Citrus Vinaigrette

- Top riced cauliflower with tofu, veggies and drizzle with the vinaigrette.

Daily Totals: 1,216 calories, 44 g protein, 149 g carbohydrates, 42 g fiber, 59 g fat, 1,248 mg sodium.

Day 10

- Chicken apple kale wraps
- Breakfast (290 calories)

  1 serving Peanut Butter-Banana Cinnamon Toast

- A.M. Snack (64 calories)

  1 cup raspberries

- Lunch (370 calories)

  1 serving Chicken & Apple Kale Wraps

  P.M. Snack (92 calories)

  1 plum

  8 almonds

- Dinner (402 calories)

1 serving Panko-Crusted Pork Chops with Asian Slaw

Daily Totals: 1,217 calories, 72 g protein, 127 g carbohydrates, 29 g fiber, 50 g fat, 1,133 mg sodium.

Day 11

Salmon & Asparagus with Lemon-Garlic Butter Sauce

Breakfast (270 calories)

- 1 serving Avocado-Egg Toast
- A.M. Snack (64 calories)

  1 cup raspberries
- Lunch (302 calories)

  1 serving Greek Kale Salad with Quinoa & Chicken
- P.M. Snack (95 calories)

  1 medium apple
- Dinner (478 calories)

  1 serving Salmon & Asparagus with Lemon-Garlic Butter Sauce

  1 cup Basic Quinoa

Meal-Prep Tip: Cook a hard-boiled egg tonight so it's ready for your P.M. Snack on Day 12.

Daily Totals: 1,209 calories, 68 g protein, 128 g carbohydrates, 28 g fiber, 50 g fat, 1,233 mg sodium.

Day 12

- Breakfast (290 calories)

  1 serving Peanut Butter-Banana Cinnamon Toast
- A.M. Snack (96 calories)

1 pancake

8 almonds

- Lunch (344 calories)

  1 1/2 cups Mexican Cabbage Soup

  2 cups mixed greens

  1 Tbsp. Citrus Vinaigrette

  2 Tbsp. sunflower seeds

  Toss greens in vinaigrette. Top with sunflower seeds.

- P.M. Snack (78 calories)

  1 hard-boiled egg, seasoned with a pinch each of salt and pepper

- Dinner (408 calories)

  1 serving Spaghetti Squash & Meatballs

Daily Totals: 1,216 calories, 60 g protein, 124 g carbohydrates, 30 g fiber, 56 g fat, 1,463 mg sodium.

Day 13

Zucchini Noodles with Avocado Pesto Shrimp

- Breakfast (264 calories)

  1 cup nonfat plain Greek yogurt

  1/4 cup muesli

  1/4 cup blueberries

- A.M. Snack (70 calories)

  2 pancakes

- Lunch (325 calories)

  1 serving Veggie & Hummus Sandwich

- P.M. Snack (95 calories)

  1 medium apple

- Dinner (446 calories)

  1 serving Zucchini Noodles with Avocado Pesto & Shrimp

Daily Totals: 1,200 calories, 68 g protein, 133 g carbohydrates, 31 g fiber, 52 g fat, 1,102 mg sodium.

Day 14

- Breakfast (270 calories)

  1 serving Avocado-Egg Toast

  A.M. Snack (70 calories)

  2 pancakes

- Lunch (378 calories)

  2 1/4 cup Tomato, Cucumber & White-Bean Salad with Basil Vinaigrette

  1 slice sprouted-grain bread, toasted and topped with 2 Tbsp. hummus

- P.M. Snack (30 calories)

  1 plum

- Dinner (458 calories)

  1 serving Fish with Coconut-Shallot Sauce

  1/2 cup Basic Quinoa

  2 cups mixed greens topped with 1 Tbsp. Citrus Vinaigrette

Daily Totals: 1,207 calories, 61 g protein, 113 g carbohydrates, 27 g fiber, 60 g fat, 1,146 mg sodium.

MEASUREMENT TABLE

▶ **LEANEST: Choose a 7-oz. portion (cooked weight) plus 2 Healthy Fat servings.**

- Fish: cod, flounder, haddock, orange roughy, grouper, tilapia, mahi mahi, tuna (yellowfin steak or canned in water), wild catfish
- Shellfish: crab, scallops, shrimp, lobster
- Game meat: deer, buffalo, elk
- Ground turkey or other meat: ≥ 98% lean
- Meatless options:
  - 14 egg whites
  - 2 cups of Egg Beaters®

▶ **LEANER: Choose a 6-oz. portion (cooked weight) plus 1 Healthy Fat serving.**

- Fish: swordfish, trout, halibut
- Chicken: breast or white meat, without skin
- Ground turkey or other meat: 95% - 97% lean
- Turkey: light meat
- Meatless options:
  - 15 oz. Mori-nu® extra-firm tofu (bean curd)
  - 2 whole eggs plus 4 egg whites

▶ **LEAN: Choose a 5-oz. portion (cooked weight) – no Healthy Fat serving added.**

- Fish: salmon, tuna (bluefin steak), farmed catfish, mackerel, herring
- Lean beef: steak, roast, ground
- Lamb
- Pork chop or pork tenderloin
- Ground turkey or other meat: 85% - 94% lean
- Chicken or turkey: dark meat
- Meatless options:
  - 15 oz. Mori-nu® firm or soft tofu (bean curd)
  - 3 whole eggs (limit to once a week)

Healthy Fat Servings

A Healthy Fat serving should contain about 5 grams of fat and less than 5 grams of carbohydrate. Add 0-2 Healthy Fat servings daily based on your Lean choices.

- 1 teaspoon of canola, flaxseed, walnut, or olive oil
- Up to 2 tablespoons of low-carbohydrate salad dressing
- 5 - 10 black or green olives
- 1 tablespoon of reduced-fat margarine
- 1½ ounces of avocado

For those requiring additional meatless choices, please refer to our Meatless Options list on the Vegetarian Information Sheet, or contact Nutrition Support at NutritionSupport@**OPTA**VIA.com.

Lean and Green Meal: "THE GREEN"

Choose three servings from our Green Options list for each of your lean and green meals. We've sorted vegetable options into lower, moderate, and higher carbohydrate levels. Each one is appropriate on the Optimal Weight 5 & 1 Plan®; the list helps you make informed food choices.

Choose 3 servings from the Green Options List:
1 serving = ½ cup vegetables (unless otherwise specified)

▶ **LOWER CARBOHYDRATE**

1 cup: collards (fresh/raw), endive, lettuce (green leaf, butterhead, iceberg, romaine), mustard greens, spinach (fresh/raw), spring mix, watercress, bok choy (raw)

½ cup: celery, cucumbers, white mushrooms, radishes, sprouts (alfalfa, mung bean), turnip greens, arugula, nopales, escarole, jalapeño (raw), Swiss chard (raw), bok choy (cooked)

▶ **MODERATE CARBOHYDRATE**

½ cup: asparagus, cabbage, cauliflower, eggplant, fennel bulb, kale, portabella mushrooms, cooked spinach, summer squash (scallop or zucchini)

▶ **HIGHER CARBOHYDRATE**

½ cup: broccoli, red cabbage, collard or mustard greens (cooked), green or wax beans, kohlrabi, okra, peppers (any color), scallions (raw), summer squash (crookneck or straightneck), tomatoes (red, ripe), turnips, spaghetti squash, hearts of palm, jicama (cooked), Swiss chard (cooked)

NOTE: All vegetables promote healthful eating. But on the Optimal Weight 5 & 1 Plan, we eliminate the highest-carbohydrate vegetables (such as carrots, corn, peas, potatoes, onions, edamame, and Brussel sprouts) to enhance your results. Once you've achieved your healthy weight, we encourage you to add all vegetables for long-term health.

CONCLUSION

This book has successfully taken you on the journey of many recipes that you can practice, prepare and embrace as a practice as you venture into maintaining a healthy and weight maintained body. These recipes are Octavia Certified and are the foods that will help you successfully achieve the goal of healthy weight loss.

Thank you for reading this far. I hope you enjoy yourself with a nice and nutritious meal that will give you that perfect shape and body you desire.

Lara Ward.

Lightning Source UK Ltd.
Milton Keynes UK
UKHW021836040621
384966UK00002B/351